Eat BETTER, Feel BETTER, LIVE BETTER

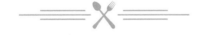

A 52-WEEK FOOD JOURNAL

NAZIMA QURESHI, RD, MPH

ROCKRIDGE
PRESS

Interior and Cover Designer: Joshua Moore
Photo Art Director/Art Manager: Sara Feinstein
Editor: Marjorie DeWitt
Production Editor: Ashley Polikoff

ISBN: 978-1-64152-625-8

THIS JOURNAL BELONGS TO

....

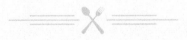

INTRODUCTION

Congratulations on the beginning of your journey to a healthier lifestyle and happier you!

A food journal is a great tool to use to achieve your goals in your journey to health and wellness. It can help with your weight loss goals and your healthy lifestyle goals. With this food journal, you'll also have the opportunity to reflect and track other aspects of your life beyond food, such as healthy habits, feelings, and exercise, if this is something you'd like to do.

Although there are many apps that track your food intake, there is something magnificent about putting pen to paper to see your goals come to life. Writing down what you eat holds you accountable to yourself. You become more aware. And you can see your eating habits and patterns clearly. This is a 52-week journal, so you can also flip back, see your progress over the course of the entire year, and know you've succeeded.

Remember, you are a wonderful individual—not after you achieve your goals, but right now. It is important to focus on your goals, but remind yourself of everything you have already achieved today. This is an exciting time in your already full life. Before you know it, you'll be making healthy eating and wellness a part of your regular routine.

> "IT DOES NOT MATTER HOW SLOWLY YOU GO SO LONG AS YOU DO NOT STOP."
> —CONFUCIUS

HOW TO USE THIS JOURNAL

This food journal is a tool to help you track what you eat, which will help you make healthier food choices. In order to get the most benefit from this journal, keep a daily log of your eating habits and all the food you eat. You may find it helpful to keep the journal with you wherever you go or make a plan to fill it out every evening.

Here are three simple steps to effectively use the journal:

1 **Fill out the Four-Week Check-In to track your progress.** Set two or three new goals and add a new healthy habit to your lifestyle every four weeks. If you aren't achieving your goals, split them into smaller goals. Tip: Set goals that are specific, measurable, and realistic.

2 **Fill out the daily food journals in as much detail as possible.** Include the amount of each food you eat and the time you eat it. Also include details such as condiments. Write down everything you consume, including snacks, beverages, and small bites.

3 **Track other health-related factors such as sleep, exercise, stress, and food cravings.** If you have a good, productive day, you'll want to remember which factors played a role. Did you exercise at all? Did you meditate? How many hours of sleep did you get? A healthy lifestyle goes far beyond what you eat.

This journal is meant to fit your personal needs, so fill out the parts that support your journey to health. If you miss a day or need to take a break from tracking, there's no need to worry—just continue where you left off.

Below is a sample entry:

4-WEEK CHECK-IN

CURRENT MEASUREMENTS

WEIGHT: _180 lbs_ ....   HIPS: ....

UPPER ARMS: ....   THIGHS: ....

CHEST: ....   CALVES: ....

WAIST: ....

WHAT ARE YOUR HOPES FOR THE NEXT FOUR WEEKS? WHAT ARE SOME GOALS YOU WOULD LIKE TO WORK TOWARD OR THINGS YOU WOULD LIKE TO IMPROVE?

I hope to feel more energized and stop eating when I'm stressed or bored. I usually snack on sweet treats because they are easily available at work and at home. I will replace these snacks with fresh fruit at home and bring healthy snacks to work. I also think exercising at least 30 minutes daily will help me boost my energy levels as well as manage my stress.

Goal: have healthy snacks twice a day
Goal: exercise at least 30 minutes daily to feel more energized

WHAT HEALTHY HABIT WOULD YOU LIKE TO ADD TO YOUR LIFESTYLE AND TRACK FOR THESE NEXT FOUR WEEKS? FEEL FREE TO CONTINUE THE OLD HABIT, TRACK A NEW HABIT, OR COMBINE THEM!

Drink at least 8 cups of water daily

Sample Food Journal Entry

DAY 1

DATE: *June 1*   HABIT: ☑

BREAKFAST	LUNCH	DINNER	SNACKS
2 egg spinach omelet Whole grain bread with tsp of butter 1 apple (9am)	1 cup mixed bean salad (black beans, red peppers, avocado, parsley) with tbsp olive oil and balsamic vinegar (12pm)	1 grilled chicken breast 1 cup roasted broccoli 1 cup quinoa with a squeeze of lemon and sea salt (5:30pm)	10 almonds (3 pm) 1 cup strawberries (7 pm)

WATER: ☑☑☑☑☑☑☑☐   FEELINGS: 😍😊😐☹😣   SLEEP: *7.5 hrs*   EXERCISE: *35 min*

CRAVINGS/RESPONSE: *I was feeling stressed at work and was craving something with crunch. Instead of reaching for chips, I had 10 almonds, and it did the trick!*

WEEKLY REFLECTIONS/NOTES

HOW DO YOU FEEL ABOUT HOW THIS WEEK WENT? WHAT CAN YOU DO TO MAKE NEXT WEEK BETTER?

I feel more energized after eating scheduled meals and snacks throughout the day. I have also swapped all of my sugary drinks with water, which is a huge win for me! Next week, I want to aim to exercise 5 days a week, as I was only able to exercise 3 days this week.   HABIT: *6* / 7

TIPS FOR WELLNESS

To achieve your goal of a healthier lifestyle, incorporate healthy habits into your day. Rather than a complete overhaul, start with one or two actions at a time until they become a habit. Here are 15 ideas to get you started:

- Be physically active for at least 30 minutes a day
- Swap sugary drinks with fruit-infused water
- Eat half a plate of raw or cooked veggies at lunch and dinner
- Pack your lunch for work instead of choosing takeout
- Grocery shop and meal plan each week
- Satisfy your craving for crunch by swapping chips for crunchy veggies or nuts
- Limit your screen time by turning off your phone notifications
- Stretch in the morning when you get out of bed—it will keep you limber!
- Choose a standing desk at work, if it is available, or get up to walk around for a few minutes every hour
- Get enough sleep
- Meditate each morning to improve your mindfulness
- Take a walk after dinner
- Avoid mindless scrolling on your phone
- Declutter your living space, one room at a time

TRACKING HEALTHY DAILY HABITS

Healthy habits are lifelong behaviors—not one-time efforts. When it comes to a healthy lifestyle, consistency and commitment are key. The power in building healthy habits is huge: you will feel better, have more energy, and eventually free up your mind to focus on other things.

This journal can be used to help you track healthy daily habits as you incorporate them into your life. Here are a few ideas, or feel free to choose one of your own.

- Walk for 30 minutes a day
- Floss
- Take a multivitamin or probiotic (or both!)
- Eat regularly scheduled meals and snacks
- Turn off all screens (including phones) two hours before bedtime
- Drink at least eight 8-ounce glasses of water each day
- Wake up earlier and watch the sunrise
- Follow a daily relaxing bedtime routine
- Read a book for 30 minutes
- Eat a healthy breakfast every morning
- Write down three things you are grateful for every day
- Tidy up an area of your living space for 10 minutes every day
- Get seven to nine hours of sleep every night
- Write in your journal
- Eat three different colorful fruits every day

LET *Food* BE THY MEDICINE AND *medicine* BE THY FOOD.

—HIPPOCRATES

GETTING STARTED

CURRENT MEASUREMENTS

WEIGHT: 120 ....

UPPER ARMS: ....

CHEST: ....

WAIST: ....

HIPS: ....

THIGHS: ....

CALVES: ....

WHAT ARE YOUR HOPES FOR THE NEXT FOUR WEEKS? WHAT ARE
SOME GOALS YOU WOULD LIKE TO WORK TOWARD OR THINGS YOU
WOULD LIKE TO IMPROVE?

....

....

....

....

....

....

....

....

WHAT HEALTHY HABIT WOULD YOU LIKE TO ADD TO YOUR LIFESTYLE
AND TRACK FOR THESE NEXT FOUR WEEKS?

....

....

....

....

....

....

....

....

....

DAY 1

DATE: HABIT: ☐

BREAKFAST	LUNCH	DINNER	SNACKS

WATER: ☐☐☐☐☐☐☐☐ FEELINGS: ☺☺☺☹☹ SLEEP: .... EXERCISE: ....
CRAVINGS/RESPONSE: ....
....

DAY 2

DATE: HABIT: ☐

BREAKFAST	LUNCH	DINNER	SNACKS

WATER: ☐☐☐☐☐☐☐☐ FEELINGS: ☺☺☺☹☹ SLEEP: .... EXERCISE: ....
CRAVINGS/RESPONSE: ....
....

DAY 3

DATE: HABIT: ☐

BREAKFAST	LUNCH	DINNER	SNACKS

WATER: ☐☐☐☐☐☐☐☐ FEELINGS: ☺☺☺☹☹ SLEEP: .... EXERCISE: ....
CRAVINGS/RESPONSE: ....
....

DAY 4

DATE: HABIT: ☐

BREAKFAST	LUNCH	DINNER	SNACKS

WATER: ☐☐☐☐☐☐☐☐ FEELINGS: ☺☺☺☹☹ SLEEP: .... EXERCISE: ....
CRAVINGS/RESPONSE: ....
....

DATE: .... HABIT: ☐

BREAKFAST	LUNCH	DINNER	SNACKS

WATER: ☐☐☐☐☐☐☐☐ FEELINGS: ☺☺☺☺☺ SLEEP: .... EXERCISE: ....

CRAVINGS/RESPONSE: ....

....

DATE: .... HABIT: ☐

BREAKFAST	LUNCH	DINNER	SNACKS

WATER: ☐☐☐☐☐☐☐☐ FEELINGS: ☺☺☺☺☺ SLEEP: .... EXERCISE: ....

CRAVINGS/RESPONSE: ....

....

DATE: .... HABIT: ☐

BREAKFAST	LUNCH	DINNER	SNACKS

WATER: ☐☐☐☐☐☐☐☐ FEELINGS: ☺☺☺☺☺ SLEEP: .... EXERCISE: ....

CRAVINGS/RESPONSE: ....

....

WEEKLY REFLECTIONS/NOTES

HOW DO YOU FEEL ABOUT HOW THIS WEEK WENT? WHAT CAN YOU DO TO MAKE NEXT WEEK BETTER?

....

....

....

.... HABIT: .... / 7

DAY 8

DATE: HABIT: ☐

BREAKFAST	LUNCH	DINNER	SNACKS

WATER: ☐☐☐☐☐☐☐☐   FEELINGS: ☺☺☺☹☹   SLEEP: ....   EXERCISE: ....

CRAVINGS/RESPONSE: ....

....

DAY 9

DATE: HABIT: ☐

BREAKFAST	LUNCH	DINNER	SNACKS

WATER: ☐☐☐☐☐☐☐☐   FEELINGS: ☺☺☺☹☹   SLEEP: ....   EXERCISE: ....

CRAVINGS/RESPONSE: ....

....

DAY 10

DATE: HABIT: ☐

BREAKFAST	LUNCH	DINNER	SNACKS

WATER: ☐☐☐☐☐☐☐☐   FEELINGS: ☺☺☺☹☹   SLEEP: ....   EXERCISE: ....

CRAVINGS/RESPONSE: ....

....

DAY 11

DATE: HABIT: ☐

BREAKFAST	LUNCH	DINNER	SNACKS

WATER: ☐☐☐☐☐☐☐☐   FEELINGS: ☺☺☺☹☹   SLEEP: ....   EXERCISE: ....

CRAVINGS/RESPONSE: ....

....

DATE: HABIT: ☐

BREAKFAST	LUNCH	DINNER	SNACKS

WATER: ☐☐☐☐☐☐☐☐ FEELINGS: ☺☺☺☹☹ SLEEP: .... EXERCISE: ....
CRAVINGS/RESPONSE: ....
....

DAY 12

DATE: HABIT: ☐

BREAKFAST	LUNCH	DINNER	SNACKS

WATER: ☐☐☐☐☐☐☐☐ FEELINGS: ☺☺☺☹☹ SLEEP: .... EXERCISE: ....
CRAVINGS/RESPONSE: ....
....

DAY 13

DATE: HABIT: ☐

BREAKFAST	LUNCH	DINNER	SNACKS

WATER: ☐☐☐☐☐☐☐☐ FEELINGS: ☺☺☺☹☹ SLEEP: .... EXERCISE: ....
CRAVINGS/RESPONSE: ....
....

DAY 14

WEEKLY REFLECTIONS/NOTES

HOW DO YOU FEEL ABOUT HOW THIS WEEK WENT? WHAT CAN YOU DO TO
MAKE NEXT WEEK BETTER?

....
....
....
.... HABIT: .... / 7

DAY 15

DATE: HABIT: ☐

BREAKFAST	LUNCH	DINNER	SNACKS

WATER: ☐☐☐☐☐☐☐☐ FEELINGS: 😊🙂😐🙁☹️ SLEEP: .... EXERCISE: ....

CRAVINGS/RESPONSE: ....

....

DAY 16

DATE: HABIT: ☐

BREAKFAST	LUNCH	DINNER	SNACKS

WATER: ☐☐☐☐☐☐☐☐ FEELINGS: 😊🙂😐🙁☹️ SLEEP: .... EXERCISE: ....

CRAVINGS/RESPONSE: ....

....

DAY 17

DATE: HABIT: ☐

BREAKFAST	LUNCH	DINNER	SNACKS

WATER: ☐☐☐☐☐☐☐☐ FEELINGS: 😊🙂😐🙁☹️ SLEEP: .... EXERCISE: ....

CRAVINGS/RESPONSE: ....

....

DAY 18

DATE: HABIT: ☐

BREAKFAST	LUNCH	DINNER	SNACKS

WATER: ☐☐☐☐☐☐☐☐ FEELINGS: 😊🙂😐🙁☹️ SLEEP: .... EXERCISE: ....

CRAVINGS/RESPONSE: ....

....

DATE: HABIT: ☐

BREAKFAST	LUNCH	DINNER	SNACKS

WATER: ☐☐☐☐☐☐☐☐ FEELINGS: ☺☺☺☹☹ SLEEP: .... EXERCISE: ....
CRAVINGS/RESPONSE: ....

DAY 19

DATE: HABIT: ☐

BREAKFAST	LUNCH	DINNER	SNACKS

WATER: ☐☐☐☐☐☐☐☐ FEELINGS: ☺☺☺☹☹ SLEEP: .... EXERCISE: ....
CRAVINGS/RESPONSE: ....

DAY 20

DATE: HABIT: ☐

BREAKFAST	LUNCH	DINNER	SNACKS

WATER: ☐☐☐☐☐☐☐☐ FEELINGS: ☺☺☺☹☹ SLEEP: .... EXERCISE: ....
CRAVINGS/RESPONSE: ....

DAY 21

WEEKLY REFLECTIONS/NOTES

HOW DO YOU FEEL ABOUT HOW THIS WEEK WENT? WHAT CAN YOU DO TO
MAKE NEXT WEEK BETTER?

....
....
....
.... HABIT: .... / 7

DAY 22

DATE: HABIT: ☐

BREAKFAST	LUNCH	DINNER	SNACKS

WATER: ☐☐☐☐☐☐☐☐   FEELINGS: ☺☺☺☹☹   SLEEP: ....   EXERCISE: ....
CRAVINGS/RESPONSE: ....
....

DAY 23

DATE: HABIT: ☐

BREAKFAST	LUNCH	DINNER	SNACKS

WATER: ☐☐☐☐☐☐☐☐   FEELINGS: ☺☺☺☹☹   SLEEP: ....   EXERCISE: ....
CRAVINGS/RESPONSE: ....
....

DAY 24

DATE: HABIT: ☐

BREAKFAST	LUNCH	DINNER	SNACKS

WATER: ☐☐☐☐☐☐☐☐   FEELINGS: ☺☺☺☹☹   SLEEP: ....   EXERCISE: ....
CRAVINGS/RESPONSE: ....
....

DAY 25

DATE: HABIT: ☐

BREAKFAST	LUNCH	DINNER	SNACKS

WATER: ☐☐☐☐☐☐☐☐   FEELINGS: ☺☺☺☹☹   SLEEP: ....   EXERCISE: ....
CRAVINGS/RESPONSE: ....
....

DATE: HABIT: ☐

BREAKFAST	LUNCH	DINNER	SNACKS

WATER: ☐☐☐☐☐☐☐☐ FEELINGS: ☺☺☺☹☹ SLEEP: .... EXERCISE: ....
CRAVINGS/RESPONSE: ....
....

DAY 26

DATE: HABIT: ☐

BREAKFAST	LUNCH	DINNER	SNACKS

WATER: ☐☐☐☐☐☐☐☐ FEELINGS: ☺☺☺☹☹ SLEEP: .... EXERCISE: ....
CRAVINGS/RESPONSE: ....
....

DAY 27

DATE: HABIT: ☐

BREAKFAST	LUNCH	DINNER	SNACKS

WATER: ☐☐☐☐☐☐☐☐ FEELINGS: ☺☺☺☹☹ SLEEP: .... EXERCISE: ....
CRAVINGS/RESPONSE: ....
....

DAY 28

WEEKLY REFLECTIONS/NOTES

HOW DO YOU FEEL ABOUT HOW THIS WEEK WENT? WHAT CAN YOU DO TO
MAKE NEXT WEEK BETTER?

....
....
....
.... HABIT: .... / 7

BEFORE *anything* ELSE, PREPARATION IS THE *key* TO SUCCESS.

-ALEXANDER GRAHAM BELL

4-WEEK CHECK-IN

CURRENT MEASUREMENTS

WEIGHT: ....

UPPER ARMS: ....

CHEST: ....

WAIST: ....

HIPS: ....

THIGHS: ....

CALVES: ....

NICE JOB!

HOW DO YOU FEEL ABOUT THE PAST FOUR WEEKS? DO YOU FEEL YOU HAVE BEEN SUCCESSFUL MEETING YOUR GOALS?

....
....
....
....
....
....

WHAT ARE YOUR HOPES FOR THE NEXT FOUR WEEKS? WHAT ARE SOME GOALS YOU WOULD LIKE TO WORK TOWARD OR THINGS YOU WOULD LIKE TO IMPROVE?

....
....
....
....
....
....

WHAT HEALTHY HABIT WOULD YOU LIKE TO ADD TO YOUR LIFESTYLE AND TRACK FOR THESE NEXT FOUR WEEKS? FEEL FREE TO CONTINUE THE OLD HABIT, TRACK A NEW HABIT, OR COMBINE THEM!

....

DAY 29

DATE: HABIT: ☐

BREAKFAST	LUNCH	DINNER	SNACKS

WATER: ☐☐☐☐☐☐☐☐ FEELINGS: ☺☺😐☹️😣 SLEEP: .... EXERCISE: ....
CRAVINGS/RESPONSE: ....
....

DAY 30

DATE: HABIT: ☐

BREAKFAST	LUNCH	DINNER	SNACKS

WATER: ☐☐☐☐☐☐☐☐ FEELINGS: ☺☺😐☹️😣 SLEEP: .... EXERCISE: ....
CRAVINGS/RESPONSE: ....
....

DAY 31

DATE: HABIT: ☐

BREAKFAST	LUNCH	DINNER	SNACKS

WATER: ☐☐☐☐☐☐☐☐ FEELINGS: ☺☺😐☹️😣 SLEEP: .... EXERCISE: ....
CRAVINGS/RESPONSE: ....
....

DAY 32

DATE: HABIT: ☐

BREAKFAST	LUNCH	DINNER	SNACKS

WATER: ☐☐☐☐☐☐☐☐ FEELINGS: ☺☺😐☹️😣 SLEEP: .... EXERCISE: ....
CRAVINGS/RESPONSE: ....
....

DATE: HABIT: ☐

BREAKFAST	LUNCH	DINNER	SNACKS

WATER: ☐☐☐☐☐☐☐☐ FEELINGS: 😊🙂😐🙁☹️ SLEEP: .... EXERCISE: ....
CRAVINGS/RESPONSE: ....
....

DAY 33

DATE: HABIT: ☐

BREAKFAST	LUNCH	DINNER	SNACKS

WATER: ☐☐☐☐☐☐☐☐ FEELINGS: 😊🙂😐🙁☹️ SLEEP: .... EXERCISE: ....
CRAVINGS/RESPONSE: ....
....

DAY 34

DATE: HABIT: ☐

BREAKFAST	LUNCH	DINNER	SNACKS

WATER: ☐☐☐☐☐☐☐☐ FEELINGS: 😊🙂😐🙁☹️ SLEEP: .... EXERCISE: ....
CRAVINGS/RESPONSE: ....
....

DAY 35

WEEKLY REFLECTIONS/NOTES

HOW DO YOU FEEL ABOUT HOW THIS WEEK WENT? WHAT CAN YOU DO TO
MAKE NEXT WEEK BETTER?

....
....
....
.... HABIT: .... / 7

DAY 36

DATE: HABIT: ☐

BREAKFAST   LUNCH   DINNER   SNACKS

WATER: ☐☐☐☐☐☐☐☐   FEELINGS: 😊🙂😐🙁☹️   SLEEP: ....   EXERCISE: ....

CRAVINGS/RESPONSE: ....

....

DAY 37

DATE: HABIT: ☐

BREAKFAST   LUNCH   DINNER   SNACKS

WATER: ☐☐☐☐☐☐☐☐   FEELINGS: 😊🙂😐🙁☹️   SLEEP: ....   EXERCISE: ....

CRAVINGS/RESPONSE: ....

....

DAY 38

DATE: HABIT: ☐

BREAKFAST   LUNCH   DINNER   SNACKS

WATER: ☐☐☐☐☐☐☐☐   FEELINGS: 😊🙂😐🙁☹️   SLEEP: ....   EXERCISE: ....

CRAVINGS/RESPONSE: ....

....

DAY 39

DATE: HABIT: ☐

BREAKFAST   LUNCH   DINNER   SNACKS

WATER: ☐☐☐☐☐☐☐☐   FEELINGS: 😊🙂😐🙁☹️   SLEEP: ....   EXERCISE: ....

CRAVINGS/RESPONSE: ....

....

DATE: .... HABIT: ☐

BREAKFAST	LUNCH	DINNER	SNACKS

WATER: ☐☐☐☐☐☐☐☐ FEELINGS: ☺☺☺☹☹ SLEEP: .... EXERCISE: ....
CRAVINGS/RESPONSE: ....
....

DAY 40

DATE: .... HABIT: ☐

BREAKFAST	LUNCH	DINNER	SNACKS

WATER: ☐☐☐☐☐☐☐☐ FEELINGS: ☺☺☺☹☹ SLEEP: .... EXERCISE: ....
CRAVINGS/RESPONSE: ....
....

DAY 41

DATE: .... HABIT: ☐

BREAKFAST	LUNCH	DINNER	SNACKS

WATER: ☐☐☐☐☐☐☐☐ FEELINGS: ☺☺☺☹☹ SLEEP: .... EXERCISE: ....
CRAVINGS/RESPONSE: ....
....

DAY 42

WEEKLY REFLECTIONS/NOTES

HOW DO YOU FEEL ABOUT HOW THIS WEEK WENT? WHAT CAN YOU DO TO
MAKE NEXT WEEK BETTER?

....
....
....
.... HABIT: .... / 7

DAY 43

DATE: .... HABIT: ☐

BREAKFAST	LUNCH	DINNER	SNACKS

WATER: ☐☐☐☐☐☐☐☐ FEELINGS: ☺☺☺☹☹ SLEEP: .... EXERCISE: ....

CRAVINGS/RESPONSE: ....
....

DAY 44

DATE: .... HABIT: ☐

BREAKFAST	LUNCH	DINNER	SNACKS

WATER: ☐☐☐☐☐☐☐☐ FEELINGS: ☺☺☺☹☹ SLEEP: .... EXERCISE: ....

CRAVINGS/RESPONSE: ....
....

DAY 45

DATE: .... HABIT: ☐

BREAKFAST	LUNCH	DINNER	SNACKS

WATER: ☐☐☐☐☐☐☐☐ FEELINGS: ☺☺☺☹☹ SLEEP: .... EXERCISE: ....

CRAVINGS/RESPONSE: ....
....

DAY 46

DATE: .... HABIT: ☐

BREAKFAST	LUNCH	DINNER	SNACKS

WATER: ☐☐☐☐☐☐☐☐ FEELINGS: ☺☺☺☹☹ SLEEP: .... EXERCISE: ....

CRAVINGS/RESPONSE: ....
....

DATE: _____ HABIT: ☐

BREAKFAST	LUNCH	DINNER	SNACKS

WATER: ☐☐☐☐☐☐☐☐ FEELINGS: 😃🙂😐😟😣 SLEEP: .... EXERCISE: ....

CRAVINGS/RESPONSE: ....

....

DAY 47

DATE: _____ HABIT: ☐

BREAKFAST	LUNCH	DINNER	SNACKS

WATER: ☐☐☐☐☐☐☐☐ FEELINGS: 😃🙂😐😟😣 SLEEP: .... EXERCISE: ....

CRAVINGS/RESPONSE: ....

....

DAY 48

DATE: _____ HABIT: ☐

BREAKFAST	LUNCH	DINNER	SNACKS

WATER: ☐☐☐☐☐☐☐☐ FEELINGS: 😃🙂😐😟😣 SLEEP: .... EXERCISE: ....

CRAVINGS/RESPONSE: ....

....

DAY 49

WEEKLY REFLECTIONS/NOTES

HOW DO YOU FEEL ABOUT HOW THIS WEEK WENT? WHAT CAN YOU DO TO MAKE NEXT WEEK BETTER?

....

....

....

.... HABIT: .... / 7

DAY 50

DATE: HABIT: ☐

BREAKFAST	LUNCH	DINNER	SNACKS

WATER: ☐☐☐☐☐☐☐☐ FEELINGS: ☺☺☺☺☺ SLEEP: .... EXERCISE: ....
CRAVINGS/RESPONSE: ....
....

DAY 51

DATE: HABIT: ☐

BREAKFAST	LUNCH	DINNER	SNACKS

WATER: ☐☐☐☐☐☐☐☐ FEELINGS: ☺☺☺☺☺ SLEEP: .... EXERCISE: ....
CRAVINGS/RESPONSE: ....
....

DAY 52

DATE: HABIT: ☐

BREAKFAST	LUNCH	DINNER	SNACKS

WATER: ☐☐☐☐☐☐☐☐ FEELINGS: ☺☺☺☺☺ SLEEP: .... EXERCISE: ....
CRAVINGS/RESPONSE: ....
....

DAY 53

DATE: HABIT: ☐

BREAKFAST	LUNCH	DINNER	SNACKS

WATER: ☐☐☐☐☐☐☐☐ FEELINGS: ☺☺☺☺☺ SLEEP: .... EXERCISE: ....
CRAVINGS/RESPONSE: ....
....

DATE: HABIT: ☐

BREAKFAST	LUNCH	DINNER	SNACKS

WATER: ☐☐☐☐☐☐☐☐ FEELINGS: ☺☺😐☹☹ SLEEP: .... EXERCISE: ....
CRAVINGS/RESPONSE: ....
....

DATE: HABIT: ☐

BREAKFAST	LUNCH	DINNER	SNACKS

WATER: ☐☐☐☐☐☐☐☐ FEELINGS: ☺☺😐☹☹ SLEEP: .... EXERCISE: ....
CRAVINGS/RESPONSE: ....
....

DATE: HABIT: ☐

BREAKFAST	LUNCH	DINNER	SNACKS

WATER: ☐☐☐☐☐☐☐☐ FEELINGS: ☺☺😐☹☹ SLEEP: .... EXERCISE: ....
CRAVINGS/RESPONSE: ....
....

WEEKLY REFLECTIONS/NOTES

HOW DO YOU FEEL ABOUT HOW THIS WEEK WENT? WHAT CAN YOU DO TO
MAKE NEXT WEEK BETTER?

....
....
....
.... HABIT: .... / 7

The GREATEST WEALTH IS *health.*

-VIRGIL

CURRENT MEASUREMENTS

WEIGHT: ....

UPPER ARMS: ....

CHEST: ....

WAIST: ....

HIPS: ....

THIGHS: ....

CALVES: ....

NICE JOB!

HOW DO YOU FEEL ABOUT THE PAST FOUR WEEKS? DO YOU FEEL
YOU HAVE BEEN SUCCESSFUL MEETING YOUR GOALS?

....

....

....

....

....

....

WHAT ARE YOUR HOPES FOR THE NEXT FOUR WEEKS? WHAT ARE
SOME GOALS YOU WOULD LIKE TO WORK TOWARD OR THINGS YOU
WOULD LIKE TO IMPROVE?

....

....

....

....

....

....

WHAT HEALTHY HABIT WOULD YOU LIKE TO ADD TO YOUR LIFESTYLE
AND TRACK FOR THESE NEXT FOUR WEEKS? FEEL FREE TO CONTINUE
THE OLD HABIT, TRACK A NEW HABIT, OR COMBINE THEM!

....

DAY 57

DATE: HABIT: ☐

BREAKFAST	LUNCH	DINNER	SNACKS

WATER: ☐☐☐☐☐☐☐☐ FEELINGS: ☺☺☺☹☹ SLEEP: .... EXERCISE: ....

CRAVINGS/RESPONSE: ....

....

DAY 58

DATE: HABIT: ☐

BREAKFAST	LUNCH	DINNER	SNACKS

WATER: ☐☐☐☐☐☐☐☐ FEELINGS: ☺☺☺☹☹ SLEEP: .... EXERCISE: ....

CRAVINGS/RESPONSE: ....

....

DAY 59

DATE: HABIT: ☐

BREAKFAST	LUNCH	DINNER	SNACKS

WATER: ☐☐☐☐☐☐☐☐ FEELINGS: ☺☺☺☹☹ SLEEP: .... EXERCISE: ....

CRAVINGS/RESPONSE: ....

....

DAY 60

DATE: HABIT: ☐

BREAKFAST	LUNCH	DINNER	SNACKS

WATER: ☐☐☐☐☐☐☐☐ FEELINGS: ☺☺☺☹☹ SLEEP: .... EXERCISE: ....

CRAVINGS/RESPONSE: ....

....

DATE: HABIT: ☐

BREAKFAST	LUNCH	DINNER	SNACKS

WATER: ☐☐☐☐☐☐☐☐   FEELINGS: ☺☺☺☹☹   SLEEP: ....   EXERCISE: ....
CRAVINGS/RESPONSE: ....
....

DATE: HABIT: ☐

BREAKFAST	LUNCH	DINNER	SNACKS

WATER: ☐☐☐☐☐☐☐☐   FEELINGS: ☺☺☺☹☹   SLEEP: ....   EXERCISE: ....
CRAVINGS/RESPONSE: ....
....

DATE: HABIT: ☐

BREAKFAST	LUNCH	DINNER	SNACKS

WATER: ☐☐☐☐☐☐☐☐   FEELINGS: ☺☺☺☹☹   SLEEP: ....   EXERCISE: ....
CRAVINGS/RESPONSE: ....
....

WEEKLY REFLECTIONS/NOTES

HOW DO YOU FEEL ABOUT HOW THIS WEEK WENT? WHAT CAN YOU DO TO
MAKE NEXT WEEK BETTER?

....
....
....
....   HABIT: .... / 7

DAY 64

DATE: HABIT: ☐

BREAKFAST   LUNCH   DINNER   SNACKS

WATER: ☐☐☐☐☐☐☐☐   FEELINGS: ☺☺☺☹☹   SLEEP: ....   EXERCISE: ....

CRAVINGS/RESPONSE: ....

....

DAY 65

DATE: HABIT: ☐

BREAKFAST   LUNCH   DINNER   SNACKS

WATER: ☐☐☐☐☐☐☐☐   FEELINGS: ☺☺☺☹☹   SLEEP: ....   EXERCISE: ....

CRAVINGS/RESPONSE: ....

....

DAY 66

DATE: HABIT: ☐

BREAKFAST   LUNCH   DINNER   SNACKS

WATER: ☐☐☐☐☐☐☐☐   FEELINGS: ☺☺☺☹☹   SLEEP: ....   EXERCISE: ....

CRAVINGS/RESPONSE: ....

....

DAY 67

DATE: HABIT: ☐

BREAKFAST   LUNCH   DINNER   SNACKS

WATER: ☐☐☐☐☐☐☐☐   FEELINGS: ☺☺☺☹☹   SLEEP: ....   EXERCISE: ....

CRAVINGS/RESPONSE: ....

....

DATE: HABIT: ☐

BREAKFAST	LUNCH	DINNER	SNACKS

WATER: ☐☐☐☐☐☐☐☐ FEELINGS: ☺☺☺☹☹ SLEEP: .... EXERCISE: ....
CRAVINGS/RESPONSE: ....
....

DAY 68

DATE: HABIT: ☐

BREAKFAST	LUNCH	DINNER	SNACKS

WATER: ☐☐☐☐☐☐☐☐ FEELINGS: ☺☺☺☹☹ SLEEP: .... EXERCISE: ....
CRAVINGS/RESPONSE: ....
....

DAY 69

DATE: HABIT: ☐

BREAKFAST	LUNCH	DINNER	SNACKS

WATER: ☐☐☐☐☐☐☐☐ FEELINGS: ☺☺☺☹☹ SLEEP: .... EXERCISE: ....
CRAVINGS/RESPONSE: ....
....

DAY 70

WEEKLY REFLECTIONS/NOTES

HOW DO YOU FEEL ABOUT HOW THIS WEEK WENT? WHAT CAN YOU DO TO
MAKE NEXT WEEK BETTER?

....
....
....
.... HABIT: .... / 7

DAY 71

DATE: HABIT: ☐

BREAKFAST	LUNCH	DINNER	SNACKS

WATER: ☐☐☐☐☐☐☐☐ FEELINGS: ☺☺☺☹☹ SLEEP: .... EXERCISE: ....

CRAVINGS/RESPONSE: ....

....

DAY 72

DATE: HABIT: ☐

BREAKFAST	LUNCH	DINNER	SNACKS

WATER: ☐☐☐☐☐☐☐☐ FEELINGS: ☺☺☺☹☹ SLEEP: .... EXERCISE: ....

CRAVINGS/RESPONSE: ....

....

DAY 73

DATE: HABIT: ☐

BREAKFAST	LUNCH	DINNER	SNACKS

WATER: ☐☐☐☐☐☐☐☐ FEELINGS: ☺☺☺☹☹ SLEEP: .... EXERCISE: ....

CRAVINGS/RESPONSE: ....

....

DAY 74

DATE: HABIT: ☐

BREAKFAST	LUNCH	DINNER	SNACKS

WATER: ☐☐☐☐☐☐☐☐ FEELINGS: ☺☺☺☹☹ SLEEP: .... EXERCISE: ....

CRAVINGS/RESPONSE: ....

....

DATE: HABIT: ☐

BREAKFAST	LUNCH	DINNER	SNACKS

WATER: ☐☐☐☐☐☐☐☐ FEELINGS: ☺☺😐🙁☹ SLEEP: .... EXERCISE: ....
CRAVINGS/RESPONSE: ....
....

DAY 75

DATE: HABIT: ☐

BREAKFAST	LUNCH	DINNER	SNACKS

WATER: ☐☐☐☐☐☐☐☐ FEELINGS: ☺☺😐🙁☹ SLEEP: .... EXERCISE: ....
CRAVINGS/RESPONSE: ....
....

DAY 76

DATE: HABIT: ☐

BREAKFAST	LUNCH	DINNER	SNACKS

WATER: ☐☐☐☐☐☐☐☐ FEELINGS: ☺☺😐🙁☹ SLEEP: .... EXERCISE: ....
CRAVINGS/RESPONSE: ....
....

DAY 77

WEEKLY REFLECTIONS/NOTES

HOW DO YOU FEEL ABOUT HOW THIS WEEK WENT? WHAT CAN YOU DO TO
MAKE NEXT WEEK BETTER?

....
....
....
.... HABIT: .... / 7

DAY 78

DATE: HABIT: ☐

BREAKFAST	LUNCH	DINNER	SNACKS

WATER: ☐☐☐☐☐☐☐☐   FEELINGS: ☺☺☺☹☹   SLEEP: ....   EXERCISE: ....
CRAVINGS/RESPONSE: ....

DAY 79

DATE: HABIT: ☐

BREAKFAST	LUNCH	DINNER	SNACKS

WATER: ☐☐☐☐☐☐☐☐   FEELINGS: ☺☺☺☹☹   SLEEP: ....   EXERCISE: ....
CRAVINGS/RESPONSE: ....

DAY 80

DATE: HABIT: ☐

BREAKFAST	LUNCH	DINNER	SNACKS

WATER: ☐☐☐☐☐☐☐☐   FEELINGS: ☺☺☺☹☹   SLEEP: ....   EXERCISE: ....
CRAVINGS/RESPONSE: ....

DAY 81

DATE: HABIT: ☐

BREAKFAST	LUNCH	DINNER	SNACKS

WATER: ☐☐☐☐☐☐☐☐   FEELINGS: ☺☺☺☹☹   SLEEP: ....   EXERCISE: ....
CRAVINGS/RESPONSE: ....

DATE: HABIT: ☐

BREAKFAST	LUNCH	DINNER	SNACKS

WATER: ☐☐☐☐☐☐☐☐ FEELINGS: ☺☺☺☹☹ SLEEP: .... EXERCISE: ....
CRAVINGS/RESPONSE: ....
....

DAY 82

DATE: HABIT: ☐

BREAKFAST	LUNCH	DINNER	SNACKS

WATER: ☐☐☐☐☐☐☐☐ FEELINGS: ☺☺☺☹☹ SLEEP: .... EXERCISE: ....
CRAVINGS/RESPONSE: ....
....

DAY 83

DATE: HABIT: ☐

BREAKFAST	LUNCH	DINNER	SNACKS

WATER: ☐☐☐☐☐☐☐☐ FEELINGS: ☺☺☺☹☹ SLEEP: .... EXERCISE: ....
CRAVINGS/RESPONSE: ....
....

DAY 84

WEEKLY REFLECTIONS/NOTES

HOW DO YOU FEEL ABOUT HOW THIS WEEK WENT? WHAT CAN YOU DO TO
MAKE NEXT WEEK BETTER?

....
....
....
.... HABIT: .... / 7

HAPPINESS
IS NOT A
goal,
IT IS A
BY-PRODUCT.

–ELEANOR ROOSEVELT

4-WEEK CHECK-IN

CURRENT MEASUREMENTS

WEIGHT: ....   HIPS: ....

UPPER ARMS: ....   THIGHS: ....

CHEST: ....   CALVES: ....

WAIST: ....

NICE JOB!

HOW DO YOU FEEL ABOUT THE PAST FOUR WEEKS? DO YOU FEEL
YOU HAVE BEEN SUCCESSFUL MEETING YOUR GOALS?

....

....

....

....

....

....

WHAT ARE YOUR HOPES FOR THE NEXT FOUR WEEKS? WHAT ARE
SOME GOALS YOU WOULD LIKE TO WORK TOWARD OR THINGS YOU
WOULD LIKE TO IMPROVE?

....

....

....

....

....

....

WHAT HEALTHY HABIT WOULD YOU LIKE TO ADD TO YOUR LIFESTYLE
AND TRACK FOR THESE NEXT FOUR WEEKS? FEEL FREE TO CONTINUE
THE OLD HABIT, TRACK A NEW HABIT, OR COMBINE THEM!

....

DAY 85

DATE: HABIT: ☐

BREAKFAST	LUNCH	DINNER	SNACKS

WATER: ☐☐☐☐☐☐☐☐ FEELINGS: ☺☺☺☹☹ SLEEP: .... EXERCISE: ....
CRAVINGS/RESPONSE: ....
....

DAY 86

DATE: HABIT: ☐

BREAKFAST	LUNCH	DINNER	SNACKS

WATER: ☐☐☐☐☐☐☐☐ FEELINGS: ☺☺☺☹☹ SLEEP: .... EXERCISE: ....
CRAVINGS/RESPONSE: ....
....

DAY 87

DATE: HABIT: ☐

BREAKFAST	LUNCH	DINNER	SNACKS

WATER: ☐☐☐☐☐☐☐☐ FEELINGS: ☺☺☺☹☹ SLEEP: .... EXERCISE: ....
CRAVINGS/RESPONSE: ....
....

DAY 88

DATE: HABIT: ☐

BREAKFAST	LUNCH	DINNER	SNACKS

WATER: ☐☐☐☐☐☐☐☐ FEELINGS: ☺☺☺☹☹ SLEEP: .... EXERCISE: ....
CRAVINGS/RESPONSE: ....
....

DATE: HABIT: ☐

BREAKFAST	LUNCH	DINNER	SNACKS

DAY 89

WATER: ☐☐☐☐☐☐☐☐   FEELINGS: ☺☺😐☹☹   SLEEP: ....   EXERCISE: ....

CRAVINGS/RESPONSE: ....

....

DATE: HABIT: ☐

BREAKFAST	LUNCH	DINNER	SNACKS

DAY 90

WATER: ☐☐☐☐☐☐☐☐   FEELINGS: ☺☺😐☹☹   SLEEP: ....   EXERCISE: ....

CRAVINGS/RESPONSE: ....

....

DATE: HABIT: ☐

BREAKFAST	LUNCH	DINNER	SNACKS

DAY 91

WATER: ☐☐☐☐☐☐☐☐   FEELINGS: ☺☺😐☹☹   SLEEP: ....   EXERCISE: ....

CRAVINGS/RESPONSE: ....

....

WEEKLY REFLECTIONS/NOTES

HOW DO YOU FEEL ABOUT HOW THIS WEEK WENT? WHAT CAN YOU DO TO
MAKE NEXT WEEK BETTER?

....

....

....

.... HABIT: .... / 7

DAY 92

DATE: HABIT: ☐

BREAKFAST   LUNCH   DINNER   SNACKS

WATER: ☐☐☐☐☐☐☐☐   FEELINGS: ☺☺☺☹☹   SLEEP: ....   EXERCISE: ....
CRAVINGS/RESPONSE: ....
....

DAY 93

DATE: HABIT: ☐

BREAKFAST   LUNCH   DINNER   SNACKS

WATER: ☐☐☐☐☐☐☐☐   FEELINGS: ☺☺☺☹☹   SLEEP: ....   EXERCISE: ....
CRAVINGS/RESPONSE: ....
....

DAY 94

DATE: HABIT: ☐

BREAKFAST   LUNCH   DINNER   SNACKS

WATER: ☐☐☐☐☐☐☐☐   FEELINGS: ☺☺☺☹☹   SLEEP: ....   EXERCISE: ....
CRAVINGS/RESPONSE: ....
....

DAY 95

DATE: HABIT: ☐

BREAKFAST   LUNCH   DINNER   SNACKS

WATER: ☐☐☐☐☐☐☐☐   FEELINGS: ☺☺☺☹☹   SLEEP: ....   EXERCISE: ....
CRAVINGS/RESPONSE: ....
....

DATE: HABIT: ☐

BREAKFAST   LUNCH   DINNER   SNACKS

WATER: ☐☐☐☐☐☐☐☐   FEELINGS: ☺☺☺☹☹   SLEEP: ....   EXERCISE: ....
CRAVINGS/RESPONSE: ....
....

DATE: HABIT: ☐

BREAKFAST   LUNCH   DINNER   SNACKS

WATER: ☐☐☐☐☐☐☐☐   FEELINGS: ☺☺☺☹☹   SLEEP: ....   EXERCISE: ....
CRAVINGS/RESPONSE: ....
....

DATE: HABIT: ☐

BREAKFAST   LUNCH   DINNER   SNACKS

WATER: ☐☐☐☐☐☐☐☐   FEELINGS: ☺☺☺☹☹   SLEEP: ....   EXERCISE: ....
CRAVINGS/RESPONSE: ....
....

WEEKLY REFLECTIONS/NOTES

HOW DO YOU FEEL ABOUT HOW THIS WEEK WENT? WHAT CAN YOU DO TO
MAKE NEXT WEEK BETTER?

....
....
....
....   HABIT: .... / 7

DAY 99

DATE: HABIT: ☐

BREAKFAST	LUNCH	DINNER	SNACKS

WATER: ☐☐☐☐☐☐☐☐ FEELINGS: ☺☺☺☹☹ SLEEP: .... EXERCISE: ....

CRAVINGS/RESPONSE: ....

....

DAY 100

DATE: HABIT: ☐

BREAKFAST	LUNCH	DINNER	SNACKS

WATER: ☐☐☐☐☐☐☐☐ FEELINGS: ☺☺☺☹☹ SLEEP: .... EXERCISE: ....

CRAVINGS/RESPONSE: ....

....

DAY 101

DATE: HABIT: ☐

BREAKFAST	LUNCH	DINNER	SNACKS

WATER: ☐☐☐☐☐☐☐☐ FEELINGS: ☺☺☺☹☹ SLEEP: .... EXERCISE: ....

CRAVINGS/RESPONSE: ....

....

DAY 102

DATE: HABIT: ☐

BREAKFAST	LUNCH	DINNER	SNACKS

WATER: ☐☐☐☐☐☐☐☐ FEELINGS: ☺☺☺☹☹ SLEEP: .... EXERCISE: ....

CRAVINGS/RESPONSE: ....

....

DATE: HABIT: ☐

BREAKFAST	LUNCH	DINNER	SNACKS

WATER: ☐☐☐☐☐☐☐☐ FEELINGS: ☺☺☺☹☹ SLEEP: .... EXERCISE: ....
CRAVINGS/RESPONSE: ....
....

DAY 103

DATE: HABIT: ☐

BREAKFAST	LUNCH	DINNER	SNACKS

WATER: ☐☐☐☐☐☐☐☐ FEELINGS: ☺☺☺☹☹ SLEEP: .... EXERCISE: ....
CRAVINGS/RESPONSE: ....
....

DAY 104

DATE: HABIT: ☐

BREAKFAST	LUNCH	DINNER	SNACKS

WATER: ☐☐☐☐☐☐☐☐ FEELINGS: ☺☺☺☹☹ SLEEP: .... EXERCISE: ....
CRAVINGS/RESPONSE: ....
....

DAY 105

WEEKLY REFLECTIONS/NOTES

HOW DO YOU FEEL ABOUT HOW THIS WEEK WENT? WHAT CAN YOU DO TO
MAKE NEXT WEEK BETTER?

....
....
....
.... HABIT: .... / 7

DAY 106

DATE: HABIT: ☐

BREAKFAST	LUNCH	DINNER	SNACKS

WATER: ☐☐☐☐☐☐☐☐ FEELINGS: ☺☺☺☹☹ SLEEP: .... EXERCISE: ....

CRAVINGS/RESPONSE: ....

....

DAY 107

DATE: HABIT: ☐

BREAKFAST	LUNCH	DINNER	SNACKS

WATER: ☐☐☐☐☐☐☐☐ FEELINGS: ☺☺☺☹☹ SLEEP: .... EXERCISE: ....

CRAVINGS/RESPONSE: ....

....

DAY 108

DATE: HABIT: ☐

BREAKFAST	LUNCH	DINNER	SNACKS

WATER: ☐☐☐☐☐☐☐☐ FEELINGS: ☺☺☺☹☹ SLEEP: .... EXERCISE: ....

CRAVINGS/RESPONSE: ....

....

DAY 109

DATE: HABIT: ☐

BREAKFAST	LUNCH	DINNER	SNACKS

WATER: ☐☐☐☐☐☐☐☐ FEELINGS: ☺☺☺☹☹ SLEEP: .... EXERCISE: ....

CRAVINGS/RESPONSE: ....

....

DATE: HABIT: □

BREAKFAST	LUNCH	DINNER	SNACKS

WATER: □□□□□□□□   FEELINGS: ☺☺☺☹☹   SLEEP: ....   EXERCISE: ....

CRAVINGS/RESPONSE: ....

....

DAY 110

DATE: HABIT: □

BREAKFAST	LUNCH	DINNER	SNACKS

WATER: □□□□□□□□   FEELINGS: ☺☺☺☹☹   SLEEP: ....   EXERCISE: ....

CRAVINGS/RESPONSE: ....

....

DAY 111

DATE: HABIT: □

BREAKFAST	LUNCH	DINNER	SNACKS

WATER: □□□□□□□□   FEELINGS: ☺☺☺☹☹   SLEEP: ....   EXERCISE: ....

CRAVINGS/RESPONSE: ....

....

DAY 112

WEEKLY REFLECTIONS/NOTES

HOW DO YOU FEEL ABOUT HOW THIS WEEK WENT? WHAT CAN YOU DO TO MAKE NEXT WEEK BETTER?

....

....

....

.... HABIT: .... / 7

THE *Best* TIME to plant a TREE WAS 20 YEARS AGO. THE SECOND BEST TIME IS *now.*

–CHINESE PROVERB

CURRENT MEASUREMENTS

WEIGHT: ....

UPPER ARMS: ....

CHEST: ....

WAIST: ....

HIPS: ....

THIGHS: ....

CALVES: ....

NICE JOB!

HOW DO YOU FEEL ABOUT THE PAST FOUR WEEKS? DO YOU FEEL
YOU HAVE BEEN SUCCESSFUL MEETING YOUR GOALS?

....

....

....

....

....

....

WHAT ARE YOUR HOPES FOR THE NEXT FOUR WEEKS? WHAT ARE
SOME GOALS YOU WOULD LIKE TO WORK TOWARD OR THINGS YOU
WOULD LIKE TO IMPROVE?

....

....

....

....

....

....

WHAT HEALTHY HABIT WOULD YOU LIKE TO ADD TO YOUR LIFESTYLE
AND TRACK FOR THESE NEXT FOUR WEEKS? FEEL FREE TO CONTINUE
THE OLD HABIT, TRACK A NEW HABIT, OR COMBINE THEM!

....

DAY 113

DATE: HABIT: ☐

BREAKFAST	LUNCH	DINNER	SNACKS

WATER: ☐☐☐☐☐☐☐☐ FEELINGS: ☺☺☺☹☹ SLEEP: .... EXERCISE: ....
CRAVINGS/RESPONSE: ....

DAY 114

DATE: HABIT: ☐

BREAKFAST	LUNCH	DINNER	SNACKS

WATER: ☐☐☐☐☐☐☐☐ FEELINGS: ☺☺☺☹☹ SLEEP: .... EXERCISE: ....
CRAVINGS/RESPONSE: ....

DAY 115

DATE: HABIT: ☐

BREAKFAST	LUNCH	DINNER	SNACKS

WATER: ☐☐☐☐☐☐☐☐ FEELINGS: ☺☺☺☹☹ SLEEP: .... EXERCISE: ....
CRAVINGS/RESPONSE: ....

DAY 116

DATE: HABIT: ☐

BREAKFAST	LUNCH	DINNER	SNACKS

WATER: ☐☐☐☐☐☐☐☐ FEELINGS: ☺☺☺☹☹ SLEEP: .... EXERCISE: ....
CRAVINGS/RESPONSE: ....

DATE: .... HABIT: ☐

BREAKFAST	LUNCH	DINNER	SNACKS

WATER: ☐☐☐☐☐☐☐☐ FEELINGS: ☺☺☺☹☹ SLEEP: .... EXERCISE: ....
CRAVINGS/RESPONSE: ....
....

DAY 117

DATE: .... HABIT: ☐

BREAKFAST	LUNCH	DINNER	SNACKS

WATER: ☐☐☐☐☐☐☐☐ FEELINGS: ☺☺☺☹☹ SLEEP: .... EXERCISE: ....
CRAVINGS/RESPONSE: ....
....

DAY 118

DATE: .... HABIT: ☐

BREAKFAST	LUNCH	DINNER	SNACKS

WATER: ☐☐☐☐☐☐☐☐ FEELINGS: ☺☺☺☹☹ SLEEP: .... EXERCISE: ....
CRAVINGS/RESPONSE: ....
....

DAY 119

WEEKLY REFLECTIONS/NOTES

HOW DO YOU FEEL ABOUT HOW THIS WEEK WENT? WHAT CAN YOU DO TO
MAKE NEXT WEEK BETTER?

....
....
....
.... HABIT: .... / 7

DAY 120

DATE: .... HABIT: ☐

BREAKFAST	LUNCH	DINNER	SNACKS

WATER: ☐☐☐☐☐☐☐☐ FEELINGS: ☺☺☺☹☹ SLEEP: .... EXERCISE: ....

CRAVINGS/RESPONSE: ....

....

DAY 121

DATE: .... HABIT: ☐

BREAKFAST	LUNCH	DINNER	SNACKS

WATER: ☐☐☐☐☐☐☐☐ FEELINGS: ☺☺☺☹☹ SLEEP: .... EXERCISE: ....

CRAVINGS/RESPONSE: ....

....

DAY 122

DATE: .... HABIT: ☐

BREAKFAST	LUNCH	DINNER	SNACKS

WATER: ☐☐☐☐☐☐☐☐ FEELINGS: ☺☺☺☹☹ SLEEP: .... EXERCISE: ....

CRAVINGS/RESPONSE: ....

....

DAY 123

DATE: .... HABIT: ☐

BREAKFAST	LUNCH	DINNER	SNACKS

WATER: ☐☐☐☐☐☐☐☐ FEELINGS: ☺☺☺☹☹ SLEEP: .... EXERCISE: ....

CRAVINGS/RESPONSE: ....

....

DATE: HABIT: ☐

BREAKFAST	LUNCH	DINNER	SNACKS

WATER: ☐☐☐☐☐☐☐☐ FEELINGS: 😊🙂😐🙁😞 SLEEP: .... EXERCISE: ....
CRAVINGS/RESPONSE: ....
....

DAY 124

DATE: HABIT: ☐

BREAKFAST	LUNCH	DINNER	SNACKS

WATER: ☐☐☐☐☐☐☐☐ FEELINGS: 😊🙂😐🙁😞 SLEEP: .... EXERCISE: ....
CRAVINGS/RESPONSE: ....
....

DAY 125

DATE: HABIT: ☐

BREAKFAST	LUNCH	DINNER	SNACKS

WATER: ☐☐☐☐☐☐☐☐ FEELINGS: 😊🙂😐🙁😞 SLEEP: .... EXERCISE: ....
CRAVINGS/RESPONSE: ....
....

DAY 126

WEEKLY REFLECTIONS/NOTES

HOW DO YOU FEEL ABOUT HOW THIS WEEK WENT? WHAT CAN YOU DO TO
MAKE NEXT WEEK BETTER?

....
....
....
.... HABIT: .... / 7

DAY 127

DATE: HABIT: ☐

BREAKFAST	LUNCH	DINNER	SNACKS

WATER: ☐☐☐☐☐☐☐☐   FEELINGS: ☺☺☺☹☹   SLEEP: ....   EXERCISE: ....
CRAVINGS/RESPONSE: ....
....

DAY 128

DATE: HABIT: ☐

BREAKFAST	LUNCH	DINNER	SNACKS

WATER: ☐☐☐☐☐☐☐☐   FEELINGS: ☺☺☺☹☹   SLEEP: ....   EXERCISE: ....
CRAVINGS/RESPONSE: ....
....

DAY 129

DATE: HABIT: ☐

BREAKFAST	LUNCH	DINNER	SNACKS

WATER: ☐☐☐☐☐☐☐☐   FEELINGS: ☺☺☺☹☹   SLEEP: ....   EXERCISE: ....
CRAVINGS/RESPONSE: ....
....

DAY 130

DATE: HABIT: ☐

BREAKFAST	LUNCH	DINNER	SNACKS

WATER: ☐☐☐☐☐☐☐☐   FEELINGS: ☺☺☺☹☹   SLEEP: ....   EXERCISE: ....
CRAVINGS/RESPONSE: ....
....

DATE: HABIT: ☐

BREAKFAST	LUNCH	DINNER	SNACKS

WATER: ☐☐☐☐☐☐☐☐ FEELINGS: ☺☺☺☹☹ SLEEP: .... EXERCISE: ....
CRAVINGS/RESPONSE: ....
....

DATE: HABIT: ☐

BREAKFAST	LUNCH	DINNER	SNACKS

WATER: ☐☐☐☐☐☐☐☐ FEELINGS: ☺☺☺☹☹ SLEEP: .... EXERCISE: ....
CRAVINGS/RESPONSE: ....
....

DATE: HABIT: ☐

BREAKFAST	LUNCH	DINNER	SNACKS

WATER: ☐☐☐☐☐☐☐☐ FEELINGS: ☺☺☺☹☹ SLEEP: .... EXERCISE: ....
CRAVINGS/RESPONSE: ....
....

WEEKLY REFLECTIONS/NOTES

HOW DO YOU FEEL ABOUT HOW THIS WEEK WENT? WHAT CAN YOU DO TO
MAKE NEXT WEEK BETTER?

....
....
....
.... HABIT: .... / 7

DATE: HABIT: ☐

BREAKFAST	LUNCH	DINNER	SNACKS

WATER: ☐☐☐☐☐☐☐☐   FEELINGS: ☺☺☺☹☹   SLEEP: ....   EXERCISE: ....
CRAVINGS/RESPONSE: ....
....

DATE: HABIT: ☐

BREAKFAST	LUNCH	DINNER	SNACKS

WATER: ☐☐☐☐☐☐☐☐   FEELINGS: ☺☺☺☹☹   SLEEP: ....   EXERCISE: ....
CRAVINGS/RESPONSE: ....
....

DATE: HABIT: ☐

BREAKFAST	LUNCH	DINNER	SNACKS

WATER: ☐☐☐☐☐☐☐☐   FEELINGS: ☺☺☺☹☹   SLEEP: ....   EXERCISE: ....
CRAVINGS/RESPONSE: ....
....

DATE: HABIT: ☐

BREAKFAST	LUNCH	DINNER	SNACKS

WATER: ☐☐☐☐☐☐☐☐   FEELINGS: ☺☺☺☹☹   SLEEP: ....   EXERCISE: ....
CRAVINGS/RESPONSE: ....
....

DATE:

BREAKFAST	LUNCH	DINNER	SNACKS

WATER: □□□□□□□□ FEELINGS: ☺☺😐☹☹ SLEEP: .... EXERCISE: ....
CRAVINGS/RESPONSE: ....

....

DAY 138

DATE: HABIT: □

BREAKFAST	LUNCH	DINNER	SNACKS

WATER: □□□□□□□□ FEELINGS: ☺☺😐☹☹ SLEEP: .... EXERCISE: ....
CRAVINGS/RESPONSE: ....

....

DAY 139

DATE: HABIT: □

BREAKFAST	LUNCH	DINNER	SNACKS

WATER: □□□□□□□□ FEELINGS: ☺☺😐☹☹ SLEEP: .... EXERCISE: ....
CRAVINGS/RESPONSE: ....

....

DAY 160

WEEKLY REFLECTIONS/NOTES

HOW DO YOU FEEL ABOUT HOW THIS WEEK WENT? WHAT CAN YOU DO TO
MAKE NEXT WEEK BETTER?

....

....

....

.... HABIT: .... / 7

One cannot *think* WELL, LOVE WELL, SLEEP WELL, IF ONE HAS NOT *dined* WELL.

–VIRGINIA WOOLF

CURRENT MEASUREMENTS

WEIGHT: ....

HIPS: ....

UPPER ARMS: ....

THIGHS: ....

CHEST: ....

CALVES: ....

WAIST: ....

NICE JOB!

HOW DO YOU FEEL ABOUT THE PAST FOUR WEEKS? DO YOU FEEL
YOU HAVE BEEN SUCCESSFUL MEETING YOUR GOALS?

....
....
....
....
....
....

WHAT ARE YOUR HOPES FOR THE NEXT FOUR WEEKS? WHAT ARE
SOME GOALS YOU WOULD LIKE TO WORK TOWARD OR THINGS YOU
WOULD LIKE TO IMPROVE?

....
....
....
....
....
....

WHAT HEALTHY HABIT WOULD YOU LIKE TO ADD TO YOUR LIFESTYLE
AND TRACK FOR THESE NEXT FOUR WEEKS? FEEL FREE TO CONTINUE
THE OLD HABIT, TRACK A NEW HABIT, OR COMBINE THEM!

....

DAY 141

DATE: HABIT: ☐

BREAKFAST	LUNCH	DINNER	SNACKS

WATER: ☐☐☐☐☐☐☐☐ FEELINGS: ☺☺☺☹☹ SLEEP: .... EXERCISE: ....
CRAVINGS/RESPONSE: ....
....

DAY 142

DATE: HABIT: ☐

BREAKFAST	LUNCH	DINNER	SNACKS

WATER: ☐☐☐☐☐☐☐☐ FEELINGS: ☺☺☺☹☹ SLEEP: .... EXERCISE: ....
CRAVINGS/RESPONSE: ....
....

DAY 143

DATE: HABIT: ☐

BREAKFAST	LUNCH	DINNER	SNACKS

WATER: ☐☐☐☐☐☐☐☐ FEELINGS: ☺☺☺☹☹ SLEEP: .... EXERCISE: ....
CRAVINGS/RESPONSE: ....
....

DAY 144

DATE: HABIT: ☐

BREAKFAST	LUNCH	DINNER	SNACKS

WATER: ☐☐☐☐☐☐☐☐ FEELINGS: ☺☺☺☹☹ SLEEP: .... EXERCISE: ....
CRAVINGS/RESPONSE: ....
....

DATE: HABIT: ☐

BREAKFAST	LUNCH	DINNER	SNACKS

WATER: ☐☐☐☐☐☐☐☐ FEELINGS: ☺☺☺☹☹ SLEEP: .... EXERCISE: ....
CRAVINGS/RESPONSE: ....
....

DAY 145

DATE: HABIT: ☐

BREAKFAST	LUNCH	DINNER	SNACKS

WATER: ☐☐☐☐☐☐☐☐ FEELINGS: ☺☺☺☹☹ SLEEP: .... EXERCISE: ....
CRAVINGS/RESPONSE: ....
....

DAY 146

DATE: HABIT: ☐

BREAKFAST	LUNCH	DINNER	SNACKS

WATER: ☐☐☐☐☐☐☐☐ FEELINGS: ☺☺☺☹☹ SLEEP: .... EXERCISE: ....
CRAVINGS/RESPONSE: ....
....

DAY 147

WEEKLY REFLECTIONS/NOTES

HOW DO YOU FEEL ABOUT HOW THIS WEEK WENT? WHAT CAN YOU DO TO
MAKE NEXT WEEK BETTER?

....
....
....
.... HABIT: .... / 7

DAY 148

DATE: _____ HABIT: ☐

BREAKFAST   LUNCH   DINNER   SNACKS

WATER: ☐☐☐☐☐☐☐☐ FEELINGS: 😊😊😐☹️☹️ SLEEP: .... EXERCISE: ....
CRAVINGS/RESPONSE: ....
....

DAY 149

DATE: _____ HABIT: ☐

BREAKFAST   LUNCH   DINNER   SNACKS

WATER: ☐☐☐☐☐☐☐☐ FEELINGS: 😊😊😐☹️☹️ SLEEP: .... EXERCISE: ....
CRAVINGS/RESPONSE: ....
....

DAY 150

DATE: _____ HABIT: ☐

BREAKFAST   LUNCH   DINNER   SNACKS

WATER: ☐☐☐☐☐☐☐☐ FEELINGS: 😊😊😐☹️☹️ SLEEP: .... EXERCISE: ....
CRAVINGS/RESPONSE: ....
....

DAY 151

DATE: _____ HABIT: ☐

BREAKFAST   LUNCH   DINNER   SNACKS

WATER: ☐☐☐☐☐☐☐☐ FEELINGS: 😊😊😐☹️☹️ SLEEP: .... EXERCISE: ....
CRAVINGS/RESPONSE: ....
....

DATE: HABIT: ☐

BREAKFAST	LUNCH	DINNER	SNACKS

WATER: ☐☐☐☐☐☐☐☐ FEELINGS: ☺☺☺☹☹ SLEEP: .... EXERCISE: ....
CRAVINGS/RESPONSE: ....
....

DAY 152

DATE: HABIT: ☐

BREAKFAST	LUNCH	DINNER	SNACKS

WATER: ☐☐☐☐☐☐☐☐ FEELINGS: ☺☺☺☹☹ SLEEP: .... EXERCISE: ....
CRAVINGS/RESPONSE: ....
....

DAY 153

DATE: HABIT: ☐

BREAKFAST	LUNCH	DINNER	SNACKS

WATER: ☐☐☐☐☐☐☐☐ FEELINGS: ☺☺☺☹☹ SLEEP: .... EXERCISE: ....
CRAVINGS/RESPONSE: ....
....

DAY 154

WEEKLY REFLECTIONS/NOTES

HOW DO YOU FEEL ABOUT HOW THIS WEEK WENT? WHAT CAN YOU DO TO
MAKE NEXT WEEK BETTER?

....
....
....
.... HABIT: .... / 7

DAY 155

DATE: HABIT: ☐

BREAKFAST	LUNCH	DINNER	SNACKS

WATER: ☐☐☐☐☐☐☐☐ FEELINGS: ☺☺☺☹☹ SLEEP: .... EXERCISE: ....
CRAVINGS/RESPONSE: ....
....

DAY 156

DATE: HABIT: ☐

BREAKFAST	LUNCH	DINNER	SNACKS

WATER: ☐☐☐☐☐☐☐☐ FEELINGS: ☺☺☺☹☹ SLEEP: .... EXERCISE: ....
CRAVINGS/RESPONSE: ....
....

DAY 157

DATE: HABIT: ☐

BREAKFAST	LUNCH	DINNER	SNACKS

WATER: ☐☐☐☐☐☐☐☐ FEELINGS: ☺☺☺☹☹ SLEEP: .... EXERCISE: ....
CRAVINGS/RESPONSE: ....
....

DAY 158

DATE: HABIT: ☐

BREAKFAST	LUNCH	DINNER	SNACKS

WATER: ☐☐☐☐☐☐☐☐ FEELINGS: ☺☺☺☹☹ SLEEP: .... EXERCISE: ....
CRAVINGS/RESPONSE: ....
....

DATE: HABIT: ☐

BREAKFAST	LUNCH	DINNER	SNACKS

WATER: ☐☐☐☐☐☐☐☐ FEELINGS: ☺☺☺☹☹ SLEEP: .... EXERCISE: ....
CRAVINGS/RESPONSE: ....
....

DAY 159

DATE: HABIT: ☐

BREAKFAST	LUNCH	DINNER	SNACKS

WATER: ☐☐☐☐☐☐☐☐ FEELINGS: ☺☺☺☹☹ SLEEP: .... EXERCISE: ....
CRAVINGS/RESPONSE: ....
....

DAY 160

DATE: HABIT: ☐

BREAKFAST	LUNCH	DINNER	SNACKS

WATER: ☐☐☐☐☐☐☐☐ FEELINGS: ☺☺☺☹☹ SLEEP: .... EXERCISE: ....
CRAVINGS/RESPONSE: ....
....

DAY 161

WEEKLY REFLECTIONS/NOTES

HOW DO YOU FEEL ABOUT HOW THIS WEEK WENT? WHAT CAN YOU DO TO
MAKE NEXT WEEK BETTER?

....
....
....
.... HABIT: .... / 7

DAY 162

DATE: HABIT: ☐

BREAKFAST	LUNCH	DINNER	SNACKS

WATER: ☐☐☐☐☐☐☐☐   FEELINGS: ☺☺☺☹☹   SLEEP: ....   EXERCISE: ....
CRAVINGS/RESPONSE: ....
....

DAY 163

DATE: HABIT: ☐

BREAKFAST	LUNCH	DINNER	SNACKS

WATER: ☐☐☐☐☐☐☐☐   FEELINGS: ☺☺☺☹☹   SLEEP: ....   EXERCISE: ....
CRAVINGS/RESPONSE: ....
....

DAY 164

DATE: HABIT: ☐

BREAKFAST	LUNCH	DINNER	SNACKS

WATER: ☐☐☐☐☐☐☐☐   FEELINGS: ☺☺☺☹☹   SLEEP: ....   EXERCISE: ....
CRAVINGS/RESPONSE: ....
....

DAY 165

DATE: HABIT: ☐

BREAKFAST	LUNCH	DINNER	SNACKS

WATER: ☐☐☐☐☐☐☐☐   FEELINGS: ☺☺☺☹☹   SLEEP: ....   EXERCISE: ....
CRAVINGS/RESPONSE: ....
....

DATE: HABIT: ☐

BREAKFAST	LUNCH	DINNER	SNACKS

WATER: ☐☐☐☐☐☐☐☐ FEELINGS: ☺☺☺☹☹ SLEEP: .... EXERCISE: ....
CRAVINGS/RESPONSE: ....
....

DATE: HABIT: ☐

BREAKFAST	LUNCH	DINNER	SNACKS

WATER: ☐☐☐☐☐☐☐☐ FEELINGS: ☺☺☺☹☹ SLEEP: .... EXERCISE: ....
CRAVINGS/RESPONSE: ....
....

DATE: HABIT: ☐

BREAKFAST	LUNCH	DINNER	SNACKS

WATER: ☐☐☐☐☐☐☐☐ FEELINGS: ☺☺☺☹☹ SLEEP: .... EXERCISE: ....
CRAVINGS/RESPONSE: ....
....

WEEKLY REFLECTIONS/NOTES

HOW DO YOU FEEL ABOUT HOW THIS WEEK WENT? WHAT CAN YOU DO TO
MAKE NEXT WEEK BETTER?

....
....
....
.... HABIT: .... / 7

Success

IS THE SUM OF

SMALL EFFORTS—
REPEATED
DAY IN (and)
DAY OUT.

–ROBERT COLLIER

4-WEEK CHECK-IN

CURRENT MEASUREMENTS

WEIGHT: ....

UPPER ARMS: ....

CHEST: ....

WAIST: ....

HIPS: ....

THIGHS: ....

CALVES: ....

NICE JOB!

HOW DO YOU FEEL ABOUT THE PAST FOUR WEEKS? DO YOU FEEL
YOU HAVE BEEN SUCCESSFUL MEETING YOUR GOALS?

....

....

....

....

....

....

WHAT ARE YOUR HOPES FOR THE NEXT FOUR WEEKS? WHAT ARE
SOME GOALS YOU WOULD LIKE TO WORK TOWARD OR THINGS YOU
WOULD LIKE TO IMPROVE?

....

....

....

....

....

....

WHAT HEALTHY HABIT WOULD YOU LIKE TO ADD TO YOUR LIFESTYLE
AND TRACK FOR THESE NEXT FOUR WEEKS? FEEL FREE TO CONTINUE
THE OLD HABIT, TRACK A NEW HABIT, OR COMBINE THEM!

....

DAY 169

DATE: HABIT: ☐

BREAKFAST	LUNCH	DINNER	SNACKS

WATER: ☐☐☐☐☐☐☐☐ FEELINGS: ☺☺😐☹☹ SLEEP: .... EXERCISE: ....
CRAVINGS/RESPONSE: ....
....

DAY 170

DATE: HABIT: ☐

BREAKFAST	LUNCH	DINNER	SNACKS

WATER: ☐☐☐☐☐☐☐☐ FEELINGS: ☺☺😐☹☹ SLEEP: .... EXERCISE: ....
CRAVINGS/RESPONSE: ....
....

DAY 171

DATE: HABIT: ☐

BREAKFAST	LUNCH	DINNER	SNACKS

WATER: ☐☐☐☐☐☐☐☐ FEELINGS: ☺☺😐☹☹ SLEEP: .... EXERCISE: ....
CRAVINGS/RESPONSE: ....
....

DAY 172

DATE: HABIT: ☐

BREAKFAST	LUNCH	DINNER	SNACKS

WATER: ☐☐☐☐☐☐☐☐ FEELINGS: ☺☺😐☹☹ SLEEP: .... EXERCISE: ....
CRAVINGS/RESPONSE: ....
....

DATE: HABIT: ☐

BREAKFAST	LUNCH	DINNER	SNACKS

WATER: ☐☐☐☐☐☐☐☐   FEELINGS: ☺☺☺☹☹   SLEEP: ....   EXERCISE: ....
CRAVINGS/RESPONSE: ....
....

DATE: HABIT: ☐

BREAKFAST	LUNCH	DINNER	SNACKS

WATER: ☐☐☐☐☐☐☐☐   FEELINGS: ☺☺☺☹☹   SLEEP: ....   EXERCISE: ....
CRAVINGS/RESPONSE: ....
....

DATE: HABIT: ☐

BREAKFAST	LUNCH	DINNER	SNACKS

WATER: ☐☐☐☐☐☐☐☐   FEELINGS: ☺☺☺☹☹   SLEEP: ....   EXERCISE: ....
CRAVINGS/RESPONSE: ....
....

WEEKLY REFLECTIONS/NOTES

HOW DO YOU FEEL ABOUT HOW THIS WEEK WENT? WHAT CAN YOU DO TO
MAKE NEXT WEEK BETTER?

....
....
....
....   HABIT: .... / 7

DATE: HABIT: ☐

BREAKFAST	LUNCH	DINNER	SNACKS

WATER: ☐☐☐☐☐☐☐☐ FEELINGS: ☺☺☺☹☹ SLEEP: .... EXERCISE: ....
CRAVINGS/RESPONSE: ....
....

DATE: HABIT: ☐

BREAKFAST	LUNCH	DINNER	SNACKS

WATER: ☐☐☐☐☐☐☐☐ FEELINGS: ☺☺☺☹☹ SLEEP: .... EXERCISE: ....
CRAVINGS/RESPONSE: ....
....

DATE: HABIT: ☐

BREAKFAST	LUNCH	DINNER	SNACKS

WATER: ☐☐☐☐☐☐☐☐ FEELINGS: ☺☺☺☹☹ SLEEP: .... EXERCISE: ....
CRAVINGS/RESPONSE: ....
....

DATE: HABIT: ☐

BREAKFAST	LUNCH	DINNER	SNACKS

WATER: ☐☐☐☐☐☐☐☐ FEELINGS: ☺☺☺☹☹ SLEEP: .... EXERCISE: ....
CRAVINGS/RESPONSE: ....
....

DATE: _____ HABIT: ☐

BREAKFAST	LUNCH	DINNER	SNACKS

WATER: ☐☐☐☐☐☐☐☐ FEELINGS: 😊🙂😐😕☹️ SLEEP: .... EXERCISE: ....

CRAVINGS/RESPONSE: ....

....

DATE: _____ HABIT: ☐

BREAKFAST	LUNCH	DINNER	SNACKS

WATER: ☐☐☐☐☐☐☐☐ FEELINGS: 😊🙂😐😕☹️ SLEEP: .... EXERCISE: ....

CRAVINGS/RESPONSE: ....

....

DATE: _____ HABIT: ☐

BREAKFAST	LUNCH	DINNER	SNACKS

WATER: ☐☐☐☐☐☐☐☐ FEELINGS: 😊🙂😐😕☹️ SLEEP: .... EXERCISE: ....

CRAVINGS/RESPONSE: ....

....

WEEKLY REFLECTIONS/NOTES

HOW DO YOU FEEL ABOUT HOW THIS WEEK WENT? WHAT CAN YOU DO TO MAKE NEXT WEEK BETTER?

....

....

....

.... HABIT: .... / 7

DAY 183

DATE: .... HABIT: ☐

BREAKFAST	LUNCH	DINNER	SNACKS

WATER: ☐☐☐☐☐☐☐☐ FEELINGS: 😊🙂😐🙁☹️ SLEEP: .... EXERCISE: ....
CRAVINGS/RESPONSE: ....
....

DAY 184

DATE: .... HABIT: ☐

BREAKFAST	LUNCH	DINNER	SNACKS

WATER: ☐☐☐☐☐☐☐☐ FEELINGS: 😊🙂😐🙁☹️ SLEEP: .... EXERCISE: ....
CRAVINGS/RESPONSE: ....
....

DAY 185

DATE: .... HABIT: ☐

BREAKFAST	LUNCH	DINNER	SNACKS

WATER: ☐☐☐☐☐☐☐☐ FEELINGS: 😊🙂😐🙁☹️ SLEEP: .... EXERCISE: ....
CRAVINGS/RESPONSE: ....
....

DAY 186

DATE: .... HABIT: ☐

BREAKFAST	LUNCH	DINNER	SNACKS

WATER: ☐☐☐☐☐☐☐☐ FEELINGS: 😊🙂😐🙁☹️ SLEEP: .... EXERCISE: ....
CRAVINGS/RESPONSE: ....
....

DATE: HABIT: ☐

BREAKFAST	LUNCH	DINNER	SNACKS

WATER: ☐☐☐☐☐☐☐☐   FEELINGS: ☺☺☺☹☹   SLEEP: ....   EXERCISE: ....

CRAVINGS/RESPONSE: ....

....

DAY 187

DATE: HABIT: ☐

BREAKFAST	LUNCH	DINNER	SNACKS

WATER: ☐☐☐☐☐☐☐☐   FEELINGS: ☺☺☺☹☹   SLEEP: ....   EXERCISE: ....

CRAVINGS/RESPONSE: ....

....

DAY 188

DATE: HABIT: ☐

BREAKFAST	LUNCH	DINNER	SNACKS

WATER: ☐☐☐☐☐☐☐☐   FEELINGS: ☺☺☺☹☹   SLEEP: ....   EXERCISE: ....

CRAVINGS/RESPONSE: ....

....

DAY 189

WEEKLY REFLECTIONS/NOTES

HOW DO YOU FEEL ABOUT HOW THIS WEEK WENT? WHAT CAN YOU DO TO MAKE NEXT WEEK BETTER?

....

....

....

.... HABIT: .... / 7

DAY 190

DATE: HABIT: ☐

BREAKFAST	LUNCH	DINNER	SNACKS

WATER: ☐☐☐☐☐☐☐☐ FEELINGS: ☺☺☺☹☹ SLEEP: .... EXERCISE: ....

CRAVINGS/RESPONSE: ....

....

DAY 191

DATE: HABIT: ☐

BREAKFAST	LUNCH	DINNER	SNACKS

WATER: ☐☐☐☐☐☐☐☐ FEELINGS: ☺☺☺☹☹ SLEEP: .... EXERCISE: ....

CRAVINGS/RESPONSE: ....

....

DAY 192

DATE: HABIT: ☐

BREAKFAST	LUNCH	DINNER	SNACKS

WATER: ☐☐☐☐☐☐☐☐ FEELINGS: ☺☺☺☹☹ SLEEP: .... EXERCISE: ....

CRAVINGS/RESPONSE: ....

....

DAY 193

DATE: HABIT: ☐

BREAKFAST	LUNCH	DINNER	SNACKS

WATER: ☐☐☐☐☐☐☐☐ FEELINGS: ☺☺☺☹☹ SLEEP: .... EXERCISE: ....

CRAVINGS/RESPONSE: ....

....

DATE: HABIT: ☐

BREAKFAST	LUNCH	DINNER	SNACKS

WATER: ☐☐☐☐☐☐☐☐   FEELINGS: ☺☺☺☹☹   SLEEP: ....   EXERCISE: ....
CRAVINGS/RESPONSE: ....
....

DAY 194

DATE: HABIT: ☐

BREAKFAST	LUNCH	DINNER	SNACKS

WATER: ☐☐☐☐☐☐☐☐   FEELINGS: ☺☺☺☹☹   SLEEP: ....   EXERCISE: ....
CRAVINGS/RESPONSE: ....
....

DAY 195

DATE: HABIT: ☐

BREAKFAST	LUNCH	DINNER	SNACKS

WATER: ☐☐☐☐☐☐☐☐   FEELINGS: ☺☺☺☹☹   SLEEP: ....   EXERCISE: ....
CRAVINGS/RESPONSE: ....
....

DAY 196

WEEKLY REFLECTIONS/NOTES

HOW DO YOU FEEL ABOUT HOW THIS WEEK WENT? WHAT CAN YOU DO TO
MAKE NEXT WEEK BETTER?

....
....
....
.... HABIT: .... / 7

The *SECRET* of
GETTING AHEAD
is **GETTING**
STARTED.

–UNKNOWN

4-WEEK CHECK-IN

CURRENT MEASUREMENTS

WEIGHT: ....

UPPER ARMS: ....

CHEST: ....

WAIST: ....

HIPS: ....

THIGHS: ....

CALVES: ....

NICE JOB!

HOW DO YOU FEEL ABOUT THE PAST FOUR WEEKS? DO YOU FEEL
YOU HAVE BEEN SUCCESSFUL MEETING YOUR GOALS?

....

....

....

....

....

....

WHAT ARE YOUR HOPES FOR THE NEXT FOUR WEEKS? WHAT ARE
SOME GOALS YOU WOULD LIKE TO WORK TOWARD OR THINGS YOU
WOULD LIKE TO IMPROVE?

....

....

....

....

....

....

WHAT HEALTHY HABIT WOULD YOU LIKE TO ADD TO YOUR LIFESTYLE
AND TRACK FOR THESE NEXT FOUR WEEKS? FEEL FREE TO CONTINUE
THE OLD HABIT, TRACK A NEW HABIT, OR COMBINE THEM!

....

DAY 197

DATE: HABIT: ☐

BREAKFAST	LUNCH	DINNER	SNACKS

WATER: ☐☐☐☐☐☐☐☐ FEELINGS: 😊☺😐🙁☹ SLEEP: .... EXERCISE: ....
CRAVINGS/RESPONSE: ....
....

DAY 198

DATE: HABIT: ☐

BREAKFAST	LUNCH	DINNER	SNACKS

WATER: ☐☐☐☐☐☐☐☐ FEELINGS: 😊☺😐🙁☹ SLEEP: .... EXERCISE: ....
CRAVINGS/RESPONSE: ....
....

DAY 199

DATE: HABIT: ☐

BREAKFAST	LUNCH	DINNER	SNACKS

WATER: ☐☐☐☐☐☐☐☐ FEELINGS: 😊☺😐🙁☹ SLEEP: .... EXERCISE: ....
CRAVINGS/RESPONSE: ....
....

DAY 200

DATE: HABIT: ☐

BREAKFAST	LUNCH	DINNER	SNACKS

WATER: ☐☐☐☐☐☐☐☐ FEELINGS: 😊☺😐🙁☹ SLEEP: .... EXERCISE: ....
CRAVINGS/RESPONSE: ....
....

DATE: \qquad HABIT: ☐

BREAKFAST	LUNCH	DINNER	SNACKS

WATER: ☐☐☐☐☐☐☐☐ FEELINGS: ☺☺☺☺☹ SLEEP: .... EXERCISE: ....
CRAVINGS/RESPONSE: ....
....

\textbf{DAY 201}

DATE: \qquad HABIT: ☐

BREAKFAST	LUNCH	DINNER	SNACKS

WATER: ☐☐☐☐☐☐☐☐ FEELINGS: ☺☺☺☺☹ SLEEP: .... EXERCISE: ....
CRAVINGS/RESPONSE: ....
....

\textbf{DAY 202}

DATE: \qquad HABIT: ☐

BREAKFAST	LUNCH	DINNER	SNACKS

WATER: ☐☐☐☐☐☐☐☐ FEELINGS: ☺☺☺☺☹ SLEEP: .... EXERCISE: ....
CRAVINGS/RESPONSE: ....
....

\textbf{DAY 203}

WEEKLY REFLECTIONS/NOTES

HOW DO YOU FEEL ABOUT HOW THIS WEEK WENT? WHAT CAN YOU DO TO
MAKE NEXT WEEK BETTER?

....
....
....
.... HABIT: .... / 7

\text{73}

DAY 204

DATE: HABIT: ☐

BREAKFAST	LUNCH	DINNER	SNACKS

WATER: ☐☐☐☐☐☐☐☐ FEELINGS: ☺☺☺☹☹ SLEEP: .... EXERCISE: ....
CRAVINGS/RESPONSE: ....

DAY 205

DATE: HABIT: ☐

BREAKFAST	LUNCH	DINNER	SNACKS

WATER: ☐☐☐☐☐☐☐☐ FEELINGS: ☺☺☺☹☹ SLEEP: .... EXERCISE: ....
CRAVINGS/RESPONSE: ....

DAY 206

DATE: HABIT: ☐

BREAKFAST	LUNCH	DINNER	SNACKS

WATER: ☐☐☐☐☐☐☐☐ FEELINGS: ☺☺☺☹☹ SLEEP: .... EXERCISE: ....
CRAVINGS/RESPONSE: ....

DAY 207

DATE: HABIT: ☐

BREAKFAST	LUNCH	DINNER	SNACKS

WATER: ☐☐☐☐☐☐☐☐ FEELINGS: ☺☺☺☹☹ SLEEP: .... EXERCISE: ....
CRAVINGS/RESPONSE: ....

DATE: HABIT: ☐

BREAKFAST	LUNCH	DINNER	SNACKS

WATER: ☐☐☐☐☐☐☐☐ FEELINGS: ☺☺☺☹☹ SLEEP: .... EXERCISE: ....
CRAVINGS/RESPONSE: ....
....

DAY 208

DATE: HABIT: ☐

BREAKFAST	LUNCH	DINNER	SNACKS

WATER: ☐☐☐☐☐☐☐☐ FEELINGS: ☺☺☺☹☹ SLEEP: .... EXERCISE: ....
CRAVINGS/RESPONSE: ....
....

DAY 209

DATE: HABIT: ☐

BREAKFAST	LUNCH	DINNER	SNACKS

WATER: ☐☐☐☐☐☐☐☐ FEELINGS: ☺☺☺☹☹ SLEEP: .... EXERCISE: ....
CRAVINGS/RESPONSE: ....
....

DAY 210

WEEKLY REFLECTIONS/NOTES

HOW DO YOU FEEL ABOUT HOW THIS WEEK WENT? WHAT CAN YOU DO TO
MAKE NEXT WEEK BETTER?

....
....
....
.... HABIT: .... / 7

DAY 211

DATE: HABIT: ☐

BREAKFAST	LUNCH	DINNER	SNACKS

WATER: ☐☐☐☐☐☐☐☐ FEELINGS: 😊🙂😐🙁☹️ SLEEP: .... EXERCISE: ....
CRAVINGS/RESPONSE: ....
....

DAY 212

DATE: HABIT: ☐

BREAKFAST	LUNCH	DINNER	SNACKS

WATER: ☐☐☐☐☐☐☐☐ FEELINGS: 😊🙂😐🙁☹️ SLEEP: .... EXERCISE: ....
CRAVINGS/RESPONSE: ....
....

DAY 213

DATE: HABIT: ☐

BREAKFAST	LUNCH	DINNER	SNACKS

WATER: ☐☐☐☐☐☐☐☐ FEELINGS: 😊🙂😐🙁☹️ SLEEP: .... EXERCISE: ....
CRAVINGS/RESPONSE: ....
....

DAY 214

DATE: HABIT: ☐

BREAKFAST	LUNCH	DINNER	SNACKS

WATER: ☐☐☐☐☐☐☐☐ FEELINGS: 😊🙂😐🙁☹️ SLEEP: .... EXERCISE: ....
CRAVINGS/RESPONSE: ....
....

DATE: HABIT: ☐

BREAKFAST	LUNCH	DINNER	SNACKS

WATER: ☐☐☐☐☐☐☐☐ FEELINGS: ☺☺☺☹☹ SLEEP: .... EXERCISE: ....
CRAVINGS/RESPONSE: ....
....

DATE: HABIT: ☐

BREAKFAST	LUNCH	DINNER	SNACKS

WATER: ☐☐☐☐☐☐☐☐ FEELINGS: ☺☺☺☹☹ SLEEP: .... EXERCISE: ....
CRAVINGS/RESPONSE: ....
....

DATE: HABIT: ☐

BREAKFAST	LUNCH	DINNER	SNACKS

WATER: ☐☐☐☐☐☐☐☐ FEELINGS: ☺☺☺☹☹ SLEEP: .... EXERCISE: ....
CRAVINGS/RESPONSE: ....
....

WEEKLY REFLECTIONS/NOTES

HOW DO YOU FEEL ABOUT HOW THIS WEEK WENT? WHAT CAN YOU DO TO
MAKE NEXT WEEK BETTER?

....
....
....
.... HABIT: .... / 7

DAY 218

DATE: HABIT: ☐

BREAKFAST	LUNCH	DINNER	SNACKS

WATER: ☐☐☐☐☐☐☐☐ FEELINGS: 😊🙂😐🙁☹️ SLEEP: .... EXERCISE: ....
CRAVINGS/RESPONSE: ....
....

DAY 219

DATE: HABIT: ☐

BREAKFAST	LUNCH	DINNER	SNACKS

WATER: ☐☐☐☐☐☐☐☐ FEELINGS: 😊🙂😐🙁☹️ SLEEP: .... EXERCISE: ....
CRAVINGS/RESPONSE: ....
....

DAY 220

DATE: HABIT: ☐

BREAKFAST	LUNCH	DINNER	SNACKS

WATER: ☐☐☐☐☐☐☐☐ FEELINGS: 😊🙂😐🙁☹️ SLEEP: .... EXERCISE: ....
CRAVINGS/RESPONSE: ....
....

DAY 221

DATE: HABIT: ☐

BREAKFAST	LUNCH	DINNER	SNACKS

WATER: ☐☐☐☐☐☐☐☐ FEELINGS: 😊🙂😐🙁☹️ SLEEP: .... EXERCISE: ....
CRAVINGS/RESPONSE: ....
....

DATE: .... HABIT: ☐

BREAKFAST	LUNCH	DINNER	SNACKS

WATER: ☐☐☐☐☐☐☐☐   FEELINGS: ☺☺☺☹☹   SLEEP: ....   EXERCISE: ....
CRAVINGS/RESPONSE: ....
....

DAY 222

DATE: .... HABIT: ☐

BREAKFAST	LUNCH	DINNER	SNACKS

WATER: ☐☐☐☐☐☐☐☐   FEELINGS: ☺☺☺☹☹   SLEEP: ....   EXERCISE: ....
CRAVINGS/RESPONSE: ....
....

DAY 223

DATE: .... HABIT: ☐

BREAKFAST	LUNCH	DINNER	SNACKS

WATER: ☐☐☐☐☐☐☐☐   FEELINGS: ☺☺☺☹☹   SLEEP: ....   EXERCISE: ....
CRAVINGS/RESPONSE: ....
....

DAY 224

WEEKLY REFLECTIONS/NOTES

HOW DO YOU FEEL ABOUT HOW THIS WEEK WENT? WHAT CAN YOU DO TO
MAKE NEXT WEEK BETTER?

....
....
....
.... HABIT: .... / 7

Happiness
IS WHEN WHAT YOU
THINK,
WHAT YOU SAY, AND WHAT YOU *do*
ARE IN HARMONY.

–MAHATMA GANDHI

4-WEEK CHECK-IN

CURRENT MEASUREMENTS

WEIGHT: ....

UPPER ARMS: ....

CHEST: ....

WAIST: ....

HIPS: ....

THIGHS: ....

CALVES: ....

NICE JOB!

HOW DO YOU FEEL ABOUT THE PAST FOUR WEEKS? DO YOU FEEL
YOU HAVE BEEN SUCCESSFUL MEETING YOUR GOALS?

....

....

....

....

....

....

WHAT ARE YOUR HOPES FOR THE NEXT FOUR WEEKS? WHAT ARE
SOME GOALS YOU WOULD LIKE TO WORK TOWARD OR THINGS YOU
WOULD LIKE TO IMPROVE?

....

....

....

....

....

....

WHAT HEALTHY HABIT WOULD YOU LIKE TO ADD TO YOUR LIFESTYLE
AND TRACK FOR THESE NEXT FOUR WEEKS? FEEL FREE TO CONTINUE
THE OLD HABIT, TRACK A NEW HABIT, OR COMBINE THEM!

....

DAY 225

DATE: HABIT: ☐

BREAKFAST	LUNCH	DINNER	SNACKS

WATER: ☐☐☐☐☐☐☐☐ FEELINGS: ☺☺☺☹☹ SLEEP: .... EXERCISE: ....
CRAVINGS/RESPONSE: ....
....

DAY 226

DATE: HABIT: ☐

BREAKFAST	LUNCH	DINNER	SNACKS

WATER: ☐☐☐☐☐☐☐☐ FEELINGS: ☺☺☺☹☹ SLEEP: .... EXERCISE: ....
CRAVINGS/RESPONSE: ....
....

DAY 227

DATE: HABIT: ☐

BREAKFAST	LUNCH	DINNER	SNACKS

WATER: ☐☐☐☐☐☐☐☐ FEELINGS: ☺☺☺☹☹ SLEEP: .... EXERCISE: ....
CRAVINGS/RESPONSE: ....
....

DAY 228

DATE: HABIT: ☐

BREAKFAST	LUNCH	DINNER	SNACKS

WATER: ☐☐☐☐☐☐☐☐ FEELINGS: ☺☺☺☹☹ SLEEP: .... EXERCISE: ....
CRAVINGS/RESPONSE: ....
....

DATE: HABIT: ☐

BREAKFAST	LUNCH	DINNER	SNACKS

WATER: ☐☐☐☐☐☐☐☐ FEELINGS: 😊🙂😐🙁☹️ SLEEP: .... EXERCISE: ....
CRAVINGS/RESPONSE: ....
....

DAY 229

DATE: HABIT: ☐

BREAKFAST	LUNCH	DINNER	SNACKS

WATER: ☐☐☐☐☐☐☐☐ FEELINGS: 😊🙂😐🙁☹️ SLEEP: .... EXERCISE: ....
CRAVINGS/RESPONSE: ....
....

DAY 230

DATE: HABIT: ☐

BREAKFAST	LUNCH	DINNER	SNACKS

WATER: ☐☐☐☐☐☐☐☐ FEELINGS: 😊🙂😐🙁☹️ SLEEP: .... EXERCISE: ....
CRAVINGS/RESPONSE: ....
....

DAY 231

WEEKLY REFLECTIONS/NOTES

HOW DO YOU FEEL ABOUT HOW THIS WEEK WENT? WHAT CAN YOU DO TO
MAKE NEXT WEEK BETTER?

....
....
....
.... HABIT: .... / 7

DATE: HABIT: ☐

BREAKFAST LUNCH DINNER SNACKS

WATER: ☐☐☐☐☐☐☐☐ FEELINGS: ☺☺☺☹☹ SLEEP: .... EXERCISE: ....
CRAVINGS/RESPONSE: ....
....

DATE: HABIT: ☐

BREAKFAST LUNCH DINNER SNACKS

WATER: ☐☐☐☐☐☐☐☐ FEELINGS: ☺☺☺☹☹ SLEEP: .... EXERCISE: ....
CRAVINGS/RESPONSE: ....
....

DATE: HABIT: ☐

BREAKFAST LUNCH DINNER SNACKS

WATER: ☐☐☐☐☐☐☐☐ FEELINGS: ☺☺☺☹☹ SLEEP: .... EXERCISE: ....
CRAVINGS/RESPONSE: ....
....

DATE: HABIT: ☐

BREAKFAST LUNCH DINNER SNACKS

WATER: ☐☐☐☐☐☐☐☐ FEELINGS: ☺☺☺☹☹ SLEEP: .... EXERCISE: ....
CRAVINGS/RESPONSE: ....
....

DATE:

BREAKFAST   LUNCH   DINNER   SNACKS

WATER: ☐☐☐☐☐☐☐☐   FEELINGS: ☺☺☺☹☹   SLEEP: ....   EXERCISE: ....
CRAVINGS/RESPONSE: ....
....

DAY 236

DATE: HABIT: ☐

BREAKFAST   LUNCH   DINNER   SNACKS

WATER: ☐☐☐☐☐☐☐☐   FEELINGS: ☺☺☺☹☹   SLEEP: ....   EXERCISE: ....
CRAVINGS/RESPONSE: ....
....

DAY 237

DATE: HABIT: ☐

BREAKFAST   LUNCH   DINNER   SNACKS

WATER: ☐☐☐☐☐☐☐☐   FEELINGS: ☺☺☺☹☹   SLEEP: ....   EXERCISE: ....
CRAVINGS/RESPONSE: ....
....

DAY 238

WEEKLY REFLECTIONS/NOTES

HOW DO YOU FEEL ABOUT HOW THIS WEEK WENT? WHAT CAN YOU DO TO
MAKE NEXT WEEK BETTER?

....
....
....
.... HABIT: .... / 7

DAY 239

DATE: HABIT: ☐

BREAKFAST	LUNCH	DINNER	SNACKS

WATER: ☐☐☐☐☐☐☐☐ FEELINGS: ☺☺☺☹☹ SLEEP: .... EXERCISE: ....

CRAVINGS/RESPONSE: ....

DAY 240

DATE: HABIT: ☐

BREAKFAST	LUNCH	DINNER	SNACKS

WATER: ☐☐☐☐☐☐☐☐ FEELINGS: ☺☺☺☹☹ SLEEP: .... EXERCISE: ....

CRAVINGS/RESPONSE: ....

DAY 241

DATE: HABIT: ☐

BREAKFAST	LUNCH	DINNER	SNACKS

WATER: ☐☐☐☐☐☐☐☐ FEELINGS: ☺☺☺☹☹ SLEEP: .... EXERCISE: ....

CRAVINGS/RESPONSE: ....

DAY 242

DATE: HABIT: ☐

BREAKFAST	LUNCH	DINNER	SNACKS

WATER: ☐☐☐☐☐☐☐☐ FEELINGS: ☺☺☺☹☹ SLEEP: .... EXERCISE: ....

CRAVINGS/RESPONSE: ....

DATE: HABIT: ☐

BREAKFAST	LUNCH	DINNER	SNACKS

WATER: ☐☐☐☐☐☐☐☐ FEELINGS: ☺☺☺☺☺ SLEEP: .... EXERCISE: ....
CRAVINGS/RESPONSE: ....
....

DATE: HABIT: ☐

BREAKFAST	LUNCH	DINNER	SNACKS

WATER: ☐☐☐☐☐☐☐☐ FEELINGS: ☺☺☺☺☺ SLEEP: .... EXERCISE: ....
CRAVINGS/RESPONSE: ....
....

DATE: HABIT: ☐

BREAKFAST	LUNCH	DINNER	SNACKS

WATER: ☐☐☐☐☐☐☐☐ FEELINGS: ☺☺☺☺☺ SLEEP: .... EXERCISE: ....
CRAVINGS/RESPONSE: ....
....

WEEKLY REFLECTIONS/NOTES

HOW DO YOU FEEL ABOUT HOW THIS WEEK WENT? WHAT CAN YOU DO TO
MAKE NEXT WEEK BETTER?

....
....
....
.... HABIT: .... / 7

DAY 246

DATE: HABIT: □

BREAKFAST	LUNCH	DINNER	SNACKS

WATER: □□□□□□□□ FEELINGS: ☺☺😐☹☹ SLEEP: .... EXERCISE: ....
CRAVINGS/RESPONSE: ....
....

DAY 247

DATE: HABIT: □

BREAKFAST	LUNCH	DINNER	SNACKS

WATER: □□□□□□□□ FEELINGS: ☺☺😐☹☹ SLEEP: .... EXERCISE: ....
CRAVINGS/RESPONSE: ....
....

DAY 248

DATE: HABIT: □

BREAKFAST	LUNCH	DINNER	SNACKS

WATER: □□□□□□□□ FEELINGS: ☺☺😐☹☹ SLEEP: .... EXERCISE: ....
CRAVINGS/RESPONSE: ....
....

DAY 249

DATE: HABIT: □

BREAKFAST	LUNCH	DINNER	SNACKS

WATER: □□□□□□□□ FEELINGS: ☺☺😐☹☹ SLEEP: .... EXERCISE: ....
CRAVINGS/RESPONSE: ....
....

DATE: HABIT: ☐

BREAKFAST	LUNCH	DINNER	SNACKS

WATER: ☐☐☐☐☐☐☐☐ FEELINGS: ☺😊😐😞😣 SLEEP: .... EXERCISE: ....
CRAVINGS/RESPONSE: ....
....

DATE: HABIT: ☐

BREAKFAST	LUNCH	DINNER	SNACKS

WATER: ☐☐☐☐☐☐☐☐ FEELINGS: ☺😊😐😞😣 SLEEP: .... EXERCISE: ....
CRAVINGS/RESPONSE: ....
....

DATE: HABIT: ☐

BREAKFAST	LUNCH	DINNER	SNACKS

WATER: ☐☐☐☐☐☐☐☐ FEELINGS: ☺😊😐😞😣 SLEEP: .... EXERCISE: ....
CRAVINGS/RESPONSE: ....
....

WEEKLY REFLECTIONS/NOTES

HOW DO YOU FEEL ABOUT HOW THIS WEEK WENT? WHAT CAN YOU DO TO
MAKE NEXT WEEK BETTER?

....
....
....
.... HABIT: .... / 7

Life

IS LIKE

RIDING A BICYCLE.

TO KEEP YOUR BALANCE YOU MUST

keep MOVING.

-ALBERT EINSTEIN

4-WEEK CHECK-IN

CURRENT MEASUREMENTS

WEIGHT: ....

HIPS: ....

UPPER ARMS: ....

THIGHS: ....

CHEST: ....

CALVES: ....

WAIST: ....

NICE JOB!

HOW DO YOU FEEL ABOUT THE PAST FOUR WEEKS? DO YOU FEEL
YOU HAVE BEEN SUCCESSFUL MEETING YOUR GOALS?

....

....

....

....

....

....

WHAT ARE YOUR HOPES FOR THE NEXT FOUR WEEKS? WHAT ARE
SOME GOALS YOU WOULD LIKE TO WORK TOWARD OR THINGS YOU
WOULD LIKE TO IMPROVE?

....

....

....

....

....

....

WHAT HEALTHY HABIT WOULD YOU LIKE TO ADD TO YOUR LIFESTYLE
AND TRACK FOR THESE NEXT FOUR WEEKS? FEEL FREE TO CONTINUE
THE OLD HABIT, TRACK A NEW HABIT, OR COMBINE THEM!

....

DAY 253

DATE: HABIT: ☐

BREAKFAST	LUNCH	DINNER	SNACKS

WATER: ☐☐☐☐☐☐☐☐ FEELINGS: ☺☺☺☹☹ SLEEP: .... EXERCISE: ....
CRAVINGS/RESPONSE: ....
....

DAY 254

DATE: HABIT: ☐

BREAKFAST	LUNCH	DINNER	SNACKS

WATER: ☐☐☐☐☐☐☐☐ FEELINGS: ☺☺☺☹☹ SLEEP: .... EXERCISE: ....
CRAVINGS/RESPONSE: ....
....

DAY 255

DATE: HABIT: ☐

BREAKFAST	LUNCH	DINNER	SNACKS

WATER: ☐☐☐☐☐☐☐☐ FEELINGS: ☺☺☺☹☹ SLEEP: .... EXERCISE: ....
CRAVINGS/RESPONSE: ....
....

DAY 256

DATE: HABIT: ☐

BREAKFAST	LUNCH	DINNER	SNACKS

WATER: ☐☐☐☐☐☐☐☐ FEELINGS: ☺☺☺☹☹ SLEEP: .... EXERCISE: ....
CRAVINGS/RESPONSE: ....
....

DATE: HABIT: ☐

BREAKFAST	LUNCH	DINNER	SNACKS

WATER: ☐☐☐☐☐☐☐☐ FEELINGS: ☺☺☺☹☹ SLEEP: .... EXERCISE: ....
CRAVINGS/RESPONSE: ....
....

DATE: HABIT: ☐

BREAKFAST	LUNCH	DINNER	SNACKS

WATER: ☐☐☐☐☐☐☐☐ FEELINGS: ☺☺☺☹☹ SLEEP: .... EXERCISE: ....
CRAVINGS/RESPONSE: ....
....

DATE: HABIT: ☐

BREAKFAST	LUNCH	DINNER	SNACKS

WATER: ☐☐☐☐☐☐☐☐ FEELINGS: ☺☺☺☹☹ SLEEP: .... EXERCISE: ....
CRAVINGS/RESPONSE: ....
....

WEEKLY REFLECTIONS/NOTES

HOW DO YOU FEEL ABOUT HOW THIS WEEK WENT? WHAT CAN YOU DO TO
MAKE NEXT WEEK BETTER?

....
....
....
.... HABIT: .... / 7

DAY 260

DATE: HABIT: ☐

BREAKFAST   LUNCH   DINNER   SNACKS

WATER: ☐☐☐☐☐☐☐☐ FEELINGS: ☺☺☺☹☹ SLEEP: .... EXERCISE: ....
CRAVINGS/RESPONSE: ....
....

DAY 261

DATE: HABIT: ☐

BREAKFAST   LUNCH   DINNER   SNACKS

WATER: ☐☐☐☐☐☐☐☐ FEELINGS: ☺☺☺☹☹ SLEEP: .... EXERCISE: ....
CRAVINGS/RESPONSE: ....
....

DAY 262

DATE: HABIT: ☐

BREAKFAST   LUNCH   DINNER   SNACKS

WATER: ☐☐☐☐☐☐☐☐ FEELINGS: ☺☺☺☹☹ SLEEP: .... EXERCISE: ....
CRAVINGS/RESPONSE: ....
....

DAY 263

DATE: HABIT: ☐

BREAKFAST   LUNCH   DINNER   SNACKS

WATER: ☐☐☐☐☐☐☐☐ FEELINGS: ☺☺☺☹☹ SLEEP: .... EXERCISE: ....
CRAVINGS/RESPONSE: ....
....

DATE: HABIT: ☐

BREAKFAST	LUNCH	DINNER	SNACKS

WATER: ☐☐☐☐☐☐☐☐ FEELINGS: ☺☺☺☹☹ SLEEP: .... EXERCISE: ....

CRAVINGS/RESPONSE: ....

....

DATE: HABIT: ☐

BREAKFAST	LUNCH	DINNER	SNACKS

WATER: ☐☐☐☐☐☐☐☐ FEELINGS: ☺☺☺☹☹ SLEEP: .... EXERCISE: ....

CRAVINGS/RESPONSE: ....

....

DATE: HABIT: ☐

BREAKFAST	LUNCH	DINNER	SNACKS

WATER: ☐☐☐☐☐☐☐☐ FEELINGS: ☺☺☺☹☹ SLEEP: .... EXERCISE: ....

CRAVINGS/RESPONSE: ....

....

WEEKLY REFLECTIONS/NOTES

HOW DO YOU FEEL ABOUT HOW THIS WEEK WENT? WHAT CAN YOU DO TO MAKE NEXT WEEK BETTER?

....

....

....

.... HABIT: .... / 7

DAY 267

DATE: HABIT: ☐

BREAKFAST	LUNCH	DINNER	SNACKS

WATER: ☐☐☐☐☐☐☐☐ FEELINGS: ☺☺☺☹☹ SLEEP: .... EXERCISE: ....
CRAVINGS/RESPONSE: ....
....

DAY 268

DATE: HABIT: ☐

BREAKFAST	LUNCH	DINNER	SNACKS

WATER: ☐☐☐☐☐☐☐☐ FEELINGS: ☺☺☺☹☹ SLEEP: .... EXERCISE: ....
CRAVINGS/RESPONSE: ....
....

DAY 269

DATE: HABIT: ☐

BREAKFAST	LUNCH	DINNER	SNACKS

WATER: ☐☐☐☐☐☐☐☐ FEELINGS: ☺☺☺☹☹ SLEEP: .... EXERCISE: ....
CRAVINGS/RESPONSE: ....
....

DAY 270

DATE: HABIT: ☐

BREAKFAST	LUNCH	DINNER	SNACKS

WATER: ☐☐☐☐☐☐☐☐ FEELINGS: ☺☺☺☹☹ SLEEP: .... EXERCISE: ....
CRAVINGS/RESPONSE: ....
....

DATE: HABIT: ☐

BREAKFAST	LUNCH	DINNER	SNACKS

WATER: ☐☐☐☐☐☐☐☐ FEELINGS: 😊🙂😐🙁☹️ SLEEP: .... EXERCISE: ....
CRAVINGS/RESPONSE: ....
....

DAY 271

DATE: HABIT: ☐

BREAKFAST	LUNCH	DINNER	SNACKS

WATER: ☐☐☐☐☐☐☐☐ FEELINGS: 😊🙂😐🙁☹️ SLEEP: .... EXERCISE: ....
CRAVINGS/RESPONSE: ....
....

DAY 272

DATE: HABIT: ☐

BREAKFAST	LUNCH	DINNER	SNACKS

WATER: ☐☐☐☐☐☐☐☐ FEELINGS: 😊🙂😐🙁☹️ SLEEP: .... EXERCISE: ....
CRAVINGS/RESPONSE: ....
....

DAY 273

WEEKLY REFLECTIONS/NOTES

HOW DO YOU FEEL ABOUT HOW THIS WEEK WENT? WHAT CAN YOU DO TO
MAKE NEXT WEEK BETTER?

....
....
....
.... HABIT: .... / 7

DAY 274

DATE: HABIT: ☐

BREAKFAST	LUNCH	DINNER	SNACKS

WATER: ☐☐☐☐☐☐☐☐   FEELINGS: ☺☺☺☹☹   SLEEP: ....   EXERCISE: ....

CRAVINGS/RESPONSE: ....

DAY 275

DATE: HABIT: ☐

BREAKFAST	LUNCH	DINNER	SNACKS

WATER: ☐☐☐☐☐☐☐☐   FEELINGS: ☺☺☺☹☹   SLEEP: ....   EXERCISE: ....

CRAVINGS/RESPONSE: ....

DAY 276

DATE: HABIT: ☐

BREAKFAST	LUNCH	DINNER	SNACKS

WATER: ☐☐☐☐☐☐☐☐   FEELINGS: ☺☺☺☹☹   SLEEP: ....   EXERCISE: ....

CRAVINGS/RESPONSE: ....

DAY 277

DATE: HABIT: ☐

BREAKFAST	LUNCH	DINNER	SNACKS

WATER: ☐☐☐☐☐☐☐☐   FEELINGS: ☺☺☺☹☹   SLEEP: ....   EXERCISE: ....

CRAVINGS/RESPONSE: ....

DATE: HABIT: ☐

BREAKFAST	LUNCH	DINNER	SNACKS

WATER: ☐☐☐☐☐☐☐☐ FEELINGS: ☺☺☺☹☹ SLEEP: .... EXERCISE: ....
CRAVINGS/RESPONSE: ....

DAY 278

DATE: HABIT: ☐

BREAKFAST	LUNCH	DINNER	SNACKS

WATER: ☐☐☐☐☐☐☐☐ FEELINGS: ☺☺☺☹☹ SLEEP: .... EXERCISE: ....
CRAVINGS/RESPONSE: ....

DAY 279

DATE: HABIT: ☐

BREAKFAST	LUNCH	DINNER	SNACKS

WATER: ☐☐☐☐☐☐☐☐ FEELINGS: ☺☺☺☹☹ SLEEP: .... EXERCISE: ....
CRAVINGS/RESPONSE: ....

DAY 280

WEEKLY REFLECTIONS/NOTES

HOW DO YOU FEEL ABOUT HOW THIS WEEK WENT? WHAT CAN YOU DO TO
MAKE NEXT WEEK BETTER?

....
....
....
.... HABIT: .... / 7

TAKE CARE OF YOUR body. IT'S THE only PLACE YOU HAVE TO LIVE.

-JIM ROHN, MOTIVATIONAL SPEAKER

4-WEEK CHECK-IN

CURRENT MEASUREMENTS

WEIGHT: ....

HIPS: ....

UPPER ARMS: ....

THIGHS: ....

CHEST: ....

CALVES: ....

WAIST: ....

NICE JOB!

HOW DO YOU FEEL ABOUT THE PAST FOUR WEEKS? DO YOU FEEL
YOU HAVE BEEN SUCCESSFUL MEETING YOUR GOALS?

....

....

....

....

....

....

WHAT ARE YOUR HOPES FOR THE NEXT FOUR WEEKS? WHAT ARE
SOME GOALS YOU WOULD LIKE TO WORK TOWARD OR THINGS YOU
WOULD LIKE TO IMPROVE?

....

....

....

....

....

....

WHAT HEALTHY HABIT WOULD YOU LIKE TO ADD TO YOUR LIFESTYLE
AND TRACK FOR THESE NEXT FOUR WEEKS? FEEL FREE TO CONTINUE
THE OLD HABIT, TRACK A NEW HABIT, OR COMBINE THEM!

....

DAY 281

DATE: HABIT: ☐

BREAKFAST	LUNCH	DINNER	SNACKS

WATER: ☐☐☐☐☐☐☐☐ FEELINGS: ☺☺☺☹☹ SLEEP: .... EXERCISE: ....

CRAVINGS/RESPONSE: ....
....

DAY 282

DATE: HABIT: ☐

BREAKFAST	LUNCH	DINNER	SNACKS

WATER: ☐☐☐☐☐☐☐☐ FEELINGS: ☺☺☺☹☹ SLEEP: .... EXERCISE: ....

CRAVINGS/RESPONSE: ....
....

DAY 283

DATE: HABIT: ☐

BREAKFAST	LUNCH	DINNER	SNACKS

WATER: ☐☐☐☐☐☐☐☐ FEELINGS: ☺☺☺☹☹ SLEEP: .... EXERCISE: ....

CRAVINGS/RESPONSE: ....
....

DAY 284

DATE: HABIT: ☐

BREAKFAST	LUNCH	DINNER	SNACKS

WATER: ☐☐☐☐☐☐☐☐ FEELINGS: ☺☺☺☹☹ SLEEP: .... EXERCISE: ....

CRAVINGS/RESPONSE: ....
....

DATE: HABIT: ☐

BREAKFAST	LUNCH	DINNER	SNACKS

WATER: ☐☐☐☐☐☐☐☐   FEELINGS: 😊🙂😐🙁☹️   SLEEP: ....   EXERCISE: ....

CRAVINGS/RESPONSE: ....

....

DAY 285

DATE: HABIT: ☐

BREAKFAST	LUNCH	DINNER	SNACKS

WATER: ☐☐☐☐☐☐☐☐   FEELINGS: 😊🙂😐🙁☹️   SLEEP: ....   EXERCISE: ....

CRAVINGS/RESPONSE: ....

....

DAY 286

DATE: HABIT: ☐

BREAKFAST	LUNCH	DINNER	SNACKS

WATER: ☐☐☐☐☐☐☐☐   FEELINGS: 😊🙂😐🙁☹️   SLEEP: ....   EXERCISE: ....

CRAVINGS/RESPONSE: ....

....

DAY 287

WEEKLY REFLECTIONS/NOTES

HOW DO YOU FEEL ABOUT HOW THIS WEEK WENT? WHAT CAN YOU DO TO
MAKE NEXT WEEK BETTER?

....

....

....

.... HABIT: .... / 7

DAY 288

DATE: HABIT: ☐

BREAKFAST	LUNCH	DINNER	SNACKS

WATER: ☐☐☐☐☐☐☐☐ FEELINGS: ☺☺☺☹☹ SLEEP: .... EXERCISE: ....

CRAVINGS/RESPONSE: ....

....

DAY 289

DATE: HABIT: ☐

BREAKFAST	LUNCH	DINNER	SNACKS

WATER: ☐☐☐☐☐☐☐☐ FEELINGS: ☺☺☺☹☹ SLEEP: .... EXERCISE: ....

CRAVINGS/RESPONSE: ....

....

DAY 290

DATE: HABIT: ☐

BREAKFAST	LUNCH	DINNER	SNACKS

WATER: ☐☐☐☐☐☐☐☐ FEELINGS: ☺☺☺☹☹ SLEEP: .... EXERCISE: ....

CRAVINGS/RESPONSE: ....

....

DAY 291

DATE: HABIT: ☐

BREAKFAST	LUNCH	DINNER	SNACKS

WATER: ☐☐☐☐☐☐☐☐ FEELINGS: ☺☺☺☹☹ SLEEP: .... EXERCISE: ....

CRAVINGS/RESPONSE: ....

....

DATE: HABIT: ☐

BREAKFAST   LUNCH   DINNER   SNACKS

WATER: ☐☐☐☐☐☐☐☐ FEELINGS: ☺☺☺☺☺ SLEEP: .... EXERCISE: ....
CRAVINGS/RESPONSE: ....
....

DATE: HABIT: ☐

BREAKFAST   LUNCH   DINNER   SNACKS

WATER: ☐☐☐☐☐☐☐☐ FEELINGS: ☺☺☺☺☺ SLEEP: .... EXERCISE: ....
CRAVINGS/RESPONSE: ....
....

DATE: HABIT: ☐

BREAKFAST   LUNCH   DINNER   SNACKS

WATER: ☐☐☐☐☐☐☐☐ FEELINGS: ☺☺☺☺☺ SLEEP: .... EXERCISE: ....
CRAVINGS/RESPONSE: ....
....

WEEKLY REFLECTIONS/NOTES

HOW DO YOU FEEL ABOUT HOW THIS WEEK WENT? WHAT CAN YOU DO TO
MAKE NEXT WEEK BETTER?

....
....
....
.... HABIT: .... / 7

DAY 295

DATE: HABIT: ☐

BREAKFAST	LUNCH	DINNER	SNACKS

WATER: ☐☐☐☐☐☐☐☐   FEELINGS: ☺☺☺☹☹   SLEEP: ....   EXERCISE: ....
CRAVINGS/RESPONSE: ....
....

DAY 296

DATE: HABIT: ☐

BREAKFAST	LUNCH	DINNER	SNACKS

WATER: ☐☐☐☐☐☐☐☐   FEELINGS: ☺☺☺☹☹   SLEEP: ....   EXERCISE: ....
CRAVINGS/RESPONSE: ....
....

DAY 297

DATE: HABIT: ☐

BREAKFAST	LUNCH	DINNER	SNACKS

WATER: ☐☐☐☐☐☐☐☐   FEELINGS: ☺☺☺☹☹   SLEEP: ....   EXERCISE: ....
CRAVINGS/RESPONSE: ....
....

DAY 298

DATE: HABIT: ☐

BREAKFAST	LUNCH	DINNER	SNACKS

WATER: ☐☐☐☐☐☐☐☐   FEELINGS: ☺☺☺☹☹   SLEEP: ....   EXERCISE: ....
CRAVINGS/RESPONSE: ....
....

DATE: HABIT: ☐

BREAKFAST	LUNCH	DINNER	SNACKS

WATER: ☐☐☐☐☐☐☐☐   FEELINGS: ☺☺😐😟☹   SLEEP: ....   EXERCISE: ....
CRAVINGS/RESPONSE: ....
....

DAY 299

DATE: HABIT: ☐

BREAKFAST	LUNCH	DINNER	SNACKS

WATER: ☐☐☐☐☐☐☐☐   FEELINGS: ☺☺😐😟☹   SLEEP: ....   EXERCISE: ....
CRAVINGS/RESPONSE: ....
....

DAY 300

DATE: HABIT: ☐

BREAKFAST	LUNCH	DINNER	SNACKS

WATER: ☐☐☐☐☐☐☐☐   FEELINGS: ☺☺😐😟☹   SLEEP: ....   EXERCISE: ....
CRAVINGS/RESPONSE: ....
....

DAY 301

WEEKLY REFLECTIONS/NOTES

HOW DO YOU FEEL ABOUT HOW THIS WEEK WENT? WHAT CAN YOU DO TO
MAKE NEXT WEEK BETTER?

....
....
....
.... HABIT: .... / 7

DAY 302

DATE: HABIT: ☐

BREAKFAST	LUNCH	DINNER	SNACKS

WATER: ☐☐☐☐☐☐☐☐ FEELINGS: ☺☺☺☹☹ SLEEP: .... EXERCISE: ....
CRAVINGS/RESPONSE: ....

DAY 303

DATE: HABIT: ☐

BREAKFAST	LUNCH	DINNER	SNACKS

WATER: ☐☐☐☐☐☐☐☐ FEELINGS: ☺☺☺☹☹ SLEEP: .... EXERCISE: ....
CRAVINGS/RESPONSE: ....

DAY 304

DATE: HABIT: ☐

BREAKFAST	LUNCH	DINNER	SNACKS

WATER: ☐☐☐☐☐☐☐☐ FEELINGS: ☺☺☺☹☹ SLEEP: .... EXERCISE: ....
CRAVINGS/RESPONSE: ....

DAY 305

DATE: HABIT: ☐

BREAKFAST	LUNCH	DINNER	SNACKS

WATER: ☐☐☐☐☐☐☐☐ FEELINGS: ☺☺☺☹☹ SLEEP: .... EXERCISE: ....
CRAVINGS/RESPONSE: ....

DATE:

BREAKFAST	LUNCH	DINNER	SNACKS

WATER: ☐☐☐☐☐☐☐☐ FEELINGS: ☺☺☺☺☺ SLEEP: .... EXERCISE: ....
CRAVINGS/RESPONSE: ....
....

DAY 306

DATE: HABIT: ☐

BREAKFAST	LUNCH	DINNER	SNACKS

WATER: ☐☐☐☐☐☐☐☐ FEELINGS: ☺☺☺☺☺ SLEEP: .... EXERCISE: ....
CRAVINGS/RESPONSE: ....
....

DAY 307

DATE: HABIT: ☐

BREAKFAST	LUNCH	DINNER	SNACKS

WATER: ☐☐☐☐☐☐☐☐ FEELINGS: ☺☺☺☺☺ SLEEP: .... EXERCISE: ....
CRAVINGS/RESPONSE: ....
....

DAY 308

WEEKLY REFLECTIONS/NOTES

HOW DO YOU FEEL ABOUT HOW THIS WEEK WENT? WHAT CAN YOU DO TO MAKE NEXT WEEK BETTER?

....
....
....
.... HABIT: .... / 7

Before
HEALING OTHERS,
HEAL
YOURSELF.

–UNKNOWN

4-WEEK CHECK-IN

CURRENT MEASUREMENTS

WEIGHT: ....

UPPER ARMS: ....

CHEST: ....

WAIST: ....

HIPS: ....

THIGHS: ....

CALVES: ....

NICE JOB!

HOW DO YOU FEEL ABOUT THE PAST FOUR WEEKS? DO YOU FEEL
YOU HAVE BEEN SUCCESSFUL MEETING YOUR GOALS?

....

....

....

....

....

....

WHAT ARE YOUR HOPES FOR THE NEXT FOUR WEEKS? WHAT ARE
SOME GOALS YOU WOULD LIKE TO WORK TOWARD OR THINGS YOU
WOULD LIKE TO IMPROVE?

....

....

....

....

....

....

WHAT HEALTHY HABIT WOULD YOU LIKE TO ADD TO YOUR LIFESTYLE
AND TRACK FOR THESE NEXT FOUR WEEKS? FEEL FREE TO CONTINUE
THE OLD HABIT, TRACK A NEW HABIT, OR COMBINE THEM!

....

DAY 309

DATE: HABIT: ☐

BREAKFAST	LUNCH	DINNER	SNACKS

WATER: ☐☐☐☐☐☐☐☐   FEELINGS: ☺☺☺☹☹   SLEEP: ....   EXERCISE: ....
CRAVINGS/RESPONSE: ....
....

DAY 310

DATE: HABIT: ☐

BREAKFAST	LUNCH	DINNER	SNACKS

WATER: ☐☐☐☐☐☐☐☐   FEELINGS: ☺☺☺☹☹   SLEEP: ....   EXERCISE: ....
CRAVINGS/RESPONSE: ....
....

DAY 311

DATE: HABIT: ☐

BREAKFAST	LUNCH	DINNER	SNACKS

WATER: ☐☐☐☐☐☐☐☐   FEELINGS: ☺☺☺☹☹   SLEEP: ....   EXERCISE: ....
CRAVINGS/RESPONSE: ....
....

DAY 312

DATE: HABIT: ☐

BREAKFAST	LUNCH	DINNER	SNACKS

WATER: ☐☐☐☐☐☐☐☐   FEELINGS: ☺☺☺☹☹   SLEEP: ....   EXERCISE: ....
CRAVINGS/RESPONSE: ....
....

DATE: HABIT: ☐

BREAKFAST	LUNCH	DINNER	SNACKS

WATER: ☐☐☐☐☐☐☐☐   FEELINGS: ☺☺☺☺☺   SLEEP: ....   EXERCISE: ....
CRAVINGS/RESPONSE: ....
....

DATE: HABIT: ☐

BREAKFAST	LUNCH	DINNER	SNACKS

WATER: ☐☐☐☐☐☐☐☐   FEELINGS: ☺☺☺☺☺   SLEEP: ....   EXERCISE: ....
CRAVINGS/RESPONSE: ....
....

DATE: HABIT: ☐

BREAKFAST	LUNCH	DINNER	SNACKS

WATER: ☐☐☐☐☐☐☐☐   FEELINGS: ☺☺☺☺☺   SLEEP: ....   EXERCISE: ....
CRAVINGS/RESPONSE: ....
....

WEEKLY REFLECTIONS/NOTES

HOW DO YOU FEEL ABOUT HOW THIS WEEK WENT? WHAT CAN YOU DO TO
MAKE NEXT WEEK BETTER?

....
....
....
....   HABIT: .... / 7

DAY 316

DATE: HABIT: ☐

BREAKFAST	LUNCH	DINNER	SNACKS

WATER: ☐☐☐☐☐☐☐☐ FEELINGS: ☺☺☺☹☹ SLEEP: .... EXERCISE: ....

CRAVINGS/RESPONSE: ....

....

DAY 317

DATE: HABIT: ☐

BREAKFAST	LUNCH	DINNER	SNACKS

WATER: ☐☐☐☐☐☐☐☐ FEELINGS: ☺☺☺☹☹ SLEEP: .... EXERCISE: ....

CRAVINGS/RESPONSE: ....

....

DAY 318

DATE: HABIT: ☐

BREAKFAST	LUNCH	DINNER	SNACKS

WATER: ☐☐☐☐☐☐☐☐ FEELINGS: ☺☺☺☹☹ SLEEP: .... EXERCISE: ....

CRAVINGS/RESPONSE: ....

....

DAY 319

DATE: HABIT: ☐

BREAKFAST	LUNCH	DINNER	SNACKS

WATER: ☐☐☐☐☐☐☐☐ FEELINGS: ☺☺☺☹☹ SLEEP: .... EXERCISE: ....

CRAVINGS/RESPONSE: ....

....

DATE: HABIT: ☐

BREAKFAST	LUNCH	DINNER	SNACKS

WATER: ☐☐☐☐☐☐☐☐   FEELINGS: ☺☺☺☹☹   SLEEP: ....   EXERCISE: ....
CRAVINGS/RESPONSE: ....
....

DAY 320

DATE: HABIT: ☐

BREAKFAST	LUNCH	DINNER	SNACKS

WATER: ☐☐☐☐☐☐☐☐   FEELINGS: ☺☺☺☹☹   SLEEP: ....   EXERCISE: ....
CRAVINGS/RESPONSE: ....
....

DAY 321

DATE: HABIT: ☐

BREAKFAST	LUNCH	DINNER	SNACKS

WATER: ☐☐☐☐☐☐☐☐   FEELINGS: ☺☺☺☹☹   SLEEP: ....   EXERCISE: ....
CRAVINGS/RESPONSE: ....
....

DAY 322

WEEKLY REFLECTIONS/NOTES

HOW DO YOU FEEL ABOUT HOW THIS WEEK WENT? WHAT CAN YOU DO TO
MAKE NEXT WEEK BETTER?

....
....
....
.... HABIT: .... / 7

DAY 323

DATE: HABIT: ☐

BREAKFAST	LUNCH	DINNER	SNACKS

WATER: ☐☐☐☐☐☐☐☐ FEELINGS: 😊🙂😐🙁☹️ SLEEP: .... EXERCISE: ....
CRAVINGS/RESPONSE: ....

DAY 324

DATE: HABIT: ☐

BREAKFAST	LUNCH	DINNER	SNACKS

WATER: ☐☐☐☐☐☐☐☐ FEELINGS: 😊🙂😐🙁☹️ SLEEP: .... EXERCISE: ....
CRAVINGS/RESPONSE: ....

DAY 325

DATE: HABIT: ☐

BREAKFAST	LUNCH	DINNER	SNACKS

WATER: ☐☐☐☐☐☐☐☐ FEELINGS: 😊🙂😐🙁☹️ SLEEP: .... EXERCISE: ....
CRAVINGS/RESPONSE: ....

DAY 326

DATE: HABIT: ☐

BREAKFAST	LUNCH	DINNER	SNACKS

WATER: ☐☐☐☐☐☐☐☐ FEELINGS: 😊🙂😐🙁☹️ SLEEP: .... EXERCISE: ....
CRAVINGS/RESPONSE: ....

DATE: HABIT: ☐

BREAKFAST	LUNCH	DINNER	SNACKS

WATER: ☐☐☐☐☐☐☐☐ FEELINGS: ☺☺☺☹☹ SLEEP: .... EXERCISE: ....
CRAVINGS/RESPONSE: ....
....

DAY 327

DATE: HABIT: ☐

BREAKFAST	LUNCH	DINNER	SNACKS

WATER: ☐☐☐☐☐☐☐☐ FEELINGS: ☺☺☺☹☹ SLEEP: .... EXERCISE: ....
CRAVINGS/RESPONSE: ....
....

DAY 328

DATE: HABIT: ☐

BREAKFAST	LUNCH	DINNER	SNACKS

WATER: ☐☐☐☐☐☐☐☐ FEELINGS: ☺☺☺☹☹ SLEEP: .... EXERCISE: ....
CRAVINGS/RESPONSE: ....
....

DAY 329

WEEKLY REFLECTIONS/NOTES

HOW DO YOU FEEL ABOUT HOW THIS WEEK WENT? WHAT CAN YOU DO TO
MAKE NEXT WEEK BETTER?

....
....
....
.... HABIT: .... / 7

DAY 330

DATE: HABIT: ☐

BREAKFAST	LUNCH	DINNER	SNACKS

WATER: ☐☐☐☐☐☐☐☐ FEELINGS: ☺☺☺☺☺ SLEEP: .... EXERCISE: ....
CRAVINGS/RESPONSE: ....
....

DAY 331

DATE: HABIT: ☐

BREAKFAST	LUNCH	DINNER	SNACKS

WATER: ☐☐☐☐☐☐☐☐ FEELINGS: ☺☺☺☺☺ SLEEP: .... EXERCISE: ....
CRAVINGS/RESPONSE: ....
....

DAY 332

DATE: HABIT: ☐

BREAKFAST	LUNCH	DINNER	SNACKS

WATER: ☐☐☐☐☐☐☐☐ FEELINGS: ☺☺☺☺☺ SLEEP: .... EXERCISE: ....
CRAVINGS/RESPONSE: ....
....

DAY 333

DATE: HABIT: ☐

BREAKFAST	LUNCH	DINNER	SNACKS

WATER: ☐☐☐☐☐☐☐☐ FEELINGS: ☺☺☺☺☺ SLEEP: .... EXERCISE: ....
CRAVINGS/RESPONSE: ....
....

DATE: HABIT: ☐

BREAKFAST	LUNCH	DINNER	SNACKS

WATER: ☐☐☐☐☐☐☐☐   FEELINGS: ☺☺☺☹☹   SLEEP: ....   EXERCISE: ....
CRAVINGS/RESPONSE: ....
....

DAY 334

DATE: HABIT: ☐

BREAKFAST	LUNCH	DINNER	SNACKS

WATER: ☐☐☐☐☐☐☐☐   FEELINGS: ☺☺☺☹☹   SLEEP: ....   EXERCISE: ....
CRAVINGS/RESPONSE: ....
....

DAY 335

DATE: HABIT: ☐

BREAKFAST	LUNCH	DINNER	SNACKS

WATER: ☐☐☐☐☐☐☐☐   FEELINGS: ☺☺☺☹☹   SLEEP: ....   EXERCISE: ....
CRAVINGS/RESPONSE: ....
....

DAY 336

WEEKLY REFLECTIONS/NOTES

HOW DO YOU FEEL ABOUT HOW THIS WEEK WENT? WHAT CAN YOU DO TO
MAKE NEXT WEEK BETTER?

....
....
....
.... HABIT: .... / 7

The BEST THING

ABOUT THE *future*

IS THAT IT COMES

ONE DAY

at a time.

–ABRAHAM LINCOLN

CURRENT MEASUREMENTS

WEIGHT: ....

HIPS: ....

UPPER ARMS: ....

THIGHS: ....

CHEST: ....

CALVES: ....

WAIST: ....

NICE JOB!

HOW DO YOU FEEL ABOUT THE PAST FOUR WEEKS? DO YOU FEEL
YOU HAVE BEEN SUCCESSFUL MEETING YOUR GOALS?

....

....

....

....

....

....

WHAT ARE YOUR HOPES FOR THE NEXT FOUR WEEKS? WHAT ARE
SOME GOALS YOU WOULD LIKE TO WORK TOWARD OR THINGS YOU
WOULD LIKE TO IMPROVE?

....

....

....

....

....

....

WHAT HEALTHY HABIT WOULD YOU LIKE TO ADD TO YOUR LIFESTYLE
AND TRACK FOR THESE NEXT FOUR WEEKS? FEEL FREE TO CONTINUE
THE OLD HABIT, TRACK A NEW HABIT, OR COMBINE THEM!

....

DAY 337

DATE: HABIT: ☐

BREAKFAST	LUNCH	DINNER	SNACKS

WATER: ☐☐☐☐☐☐☐☐   FEELINGS: ☺☺☺☹☹   SLEEP: ....   EXERCISE: ....
CRAVINGS/RESPONSE: ....

DAY 338

DATE: HABIT: ☐

BREAKFAST	LUNCH	DINNER	SNACKS

WATER: ☐☐☐☐☐☐☐☐   FEELINGS: ☺☺☺☹☹   SLEEP: ....   EXERCISE: ....
CRAVINGS/RESPONSE: ....

DAY 339

DATE: HABIT: ☐

BREAKFAST	LUNCH	DINNER	SNACKS

WATER: ☐☐☐☐☐☐☐☐   FEELINGS: ☺☺☺☹☹   SLEEP: ....   EXERCISE: ....
CRAVINGS/RESPONSE: ....

DAY 340

DATE: HABIT: ☐

BREAKFAST	LUNCH	DINNER	SNACKS

WATER: ☐☐☐☐☐☐☐☐   FEELINGS: ☺☺☺☹☹   SLEEP: ....   EXERCISE: ....
CRAVINGS/RESPONSE: ....

DATE: HABIT: ☐

BREAKFAST	LUNCH	DINNER	SNACKS

WATER: ☐☐☐☐☐☐☐☐ FEELINGS: ☺☺☺☹☹ SLEEP: .... EXERCISE: ....
CRAVINGS/RESPONSE: ....
....

DAY 341

DATE: HABIT: ☐

BREAKFAST	LUNCH	DINNER	SNACKS

WATER: ☐☐☐☐☐☐☐☐ FEELINGS: ☺☺☺☹☹ SLEEP: .... EXERCISE: ....
CRAVINGS/RESPONSE: ....
....

DAY 342

DATE: HABIT: ☐

BREAKFAST	LUNCH	DINNER	SNACKS

WATER: ☐☐☐☐☐☐☐☐ FEELINGS: ☺☺☺☹☹ SLEEP: .... EXERCISE: ....
CRAVINGS/RESPONSE: ....
....

DAY 343

WEEKLY REFLECTIONS/NOTES

HOW DO YOU FEEL ABOUT HOW THIS WEEK WENT? WHAT CAN YOU DO TO
MAKE NEXT WEEK BETTER?

....
....
....
.... HABIT: .... / 7

DAY 344

DATE: HABIT: ☐

BREAKFAST	LUNCH	DINNER	SNACKS

WATER: ☐☐☐☐☐☐☐☐ FEELINGS: ☺☺☺☹☹ SLEEP: .... EXERCISE: ....
CRAVINGS/RESPONSE: ....
....

DAY 345

DATE: HABIT: ☐

BREAKFAST	LUNCH	DINNER	SNACKS

WATER: ☐☐☐☐☐☐☐☐ FEELINGS: ☺☺☺☹☹ SLEEP: .... EXERCISE: ....
CRAVINGS/RESPONSE: ....
....

DAY 346

DATE: HABIT: ☐

BREAKFAST	LUNCH	DINNER	SNACKS

WATER: ☐☐☐☐☐☐☐☐ FEELINGS: ☺☺☺☹☹ SLEEP: .... EXERCISE: ....
CRAVINGS/RESPONSE: ....
....

DAY 347

DATE: HABIT: ☐

BREAKFAST	LUNCH	DINNER	SNACKS

WATER: ☐☐☐☐☐☐☐☐ FEELINGS: ☺☺☺☹☹ SLEEP: .... EXERCISE: ....
CRAVINGS/RESPONSE: ....
....

DATE: .... HABIT: ☐

BREAKFAST	LUNCH	DINNER	SNACKS

WATER: ☐☐☐☐☐☐☐☐ FEELINGS: ☺☺☺☹☹ SLEEP: .... EXERCISE: ....

CRAVINGS/RESPONSE: ....

....

DATE: .... HABIT: ☐

BREAKFAST	LUNCH	DINNER	SNACKS

WATER: ☐☐☐☐☐☐☐☐ FEELINGS: ☺☺☺☹☹ SLEEP: .... EXERCISE: ....

CRAVINGS/RESPONSE: ....

....

DATE: .... HABIT: ☐

BREAKFAST	LUNCH	DINNER	SNACKS

WATER: ☐☐☐☐☐☐☐☐ FEELINGS: ☺☺☺☹☹ SLEEP: .... EXERCISE: ....

CRAVINGS/RESPONSE: ....

....

WEEKLY REFLECTIONS/NOTES

HOW DO YOU FEEL ABOUT HOW THIS WEEK WENT? WHAT CAN YOU DO TO MAKE NEXT WEEK BETTER?

....

....

....

.... HABIT: .... / 7

DAY 351

DATE: HABIT: ☐

BREAKFAST	LUNCH	DINNER	SNACKS

WATER: ☐☐☐☐☐☐☐☐ FEELINGS: ☺☺☺☹☹ SLEEP: .... EXERCISE: ....

CRAVINGS/RESPONSE: ....
....

DAY 352

DATE: HABIT: ☐

BREAKFAST	LUNCH	DINNER	SNACKS

WATER: ☐☐☐☐☐☐☐☐ FEELINGS: ☺☺☺☹☹ SLEEP: .... EXERCISE: ....

CRAVINGS/RESPONSE: ....
....

DAY 353

DATE: HABIT: ☐

BREAKFAST	LUNCH	DINNER	SNACKS

WATER: ☐☐☐☐☐☐☐☐ FEELINGS: ☺☺☺☹☹ SLEEP: .... EXERCISE: ....

CRAVINGS/RESPONSE: ....
....

DAY 354

DATE: HABIT: ☐

BREAKFAST	LUNCH	DINNER	SNACKS

WATER: ☐☐☐☐☐☐☐☐ FEELINGS: ☺☺☺☹☹ SLEEP: .... EXERCISE: ....

CRAVINGS/RESPONSE: ....
....

DATE: HABIT: ☐

BREAKFAST	LUNCH	DINNER	SNACKS

WATER: ☐☐☐☐☐☐☐☐   FEELINGS: ☺☺☺☹☹   SLEEP: ....   EXERCISE: ....
CRAVINGS/RESPONSE: ....
....

DAY 355

DATE: HABIT: ☐

BREAKFAST	LUNCH	DINNER	SNACKS

WATER: ☐☐☐☐☐☐☐☐   FEELINGS: ☺☺☺☹☹   SLEEP: ....   EXERCISE: ....
CRAVINGS/RESPONSE: ....
....

DAY 356

DATE: HABIT: ☐

BREAKFAST	LUNCH	DINNER	SNACKS

WATER: ☐☐☐☐☐☐☐☐   FEELINGS: ☺☺☺☹☹   SLEEP: ....   EXERCISE: ....
CRAVINGS/RESPONSE: ....
....

DAY 357

WEEKLY REFLECTIONS/NOTES

HOW DO YOU FEEL ABOUT HOW THIS WEEK WENT? WHAT CAN YOU DO TO
MAKE NEXT WEEK BETTER?

....
....
....
.... HABIT: .... / 7

DAY 358

DATE: HABIT: ☐

BREAKFAST	LUNCH	DINNER	SNACKS

WATER: ☐☐☐☐☐☐☐☐ FEELINGS: ☺☺☺☹☹ SLEEP: .... EXERCISE: ....

CRAVINGS/RESPONSE: ....

....

DAY 359

DATE: HABIT: ☐

BREAKFAST	LUNCH	DINNER	SNACKS

WATER: ☐☐☐☐☐☐☐☐ FEELINGS: ☺☺☺☹☹ SLEEP: .... EXERCISE: ....

CRAVINGS/RESPONSE: ....

....

DAY 360

DATE: HABIT: ☐

BREAKFAST	LUNCH	DINNER	SNACKS

WATER: ☐☐☐☐☐☐☐☐ FEELINGS: ☺☺☺☹☹ SLEEP: .... EXERCISE: ....

CRAVINGS/RESPONSE: ....

....

DAY 361

DATE: HABIT: ☐

BREAKFAST	LUNCH	DINNER	SNACKS

WATER: ☐☐☐☐☐☐☐☐ FEELINGS: ☺☺☺☹☹ SLEEP: .... EXERCISE: ....

CRAVINGS/RESPONSE: ....

....

DATE: HABIT: ☐

BREAKFAST	LUNCH	DINNER	SNACKS

WATER: ☐☐☐☐☐☐☐☐   FEELINGS: ☺☺☺☹☹   SLEEP: ....   EXERCISE: ....
CRAVINGS/RESPONSE: ....
....

DAY 362

DATE: HABIT: ☐

BREAKFAST	LUNCH	DINNER	SNACKS

WATER: ☐☐☐☐☐☐☐☐   FEELINGS: ☺☺☺☹☹   SLEEP: ....   EXERCISE: ....
CRAVINGS/RESPONSE: ....
....

DAY 363

DATE: HABIT: ☐

BREAKFAST	LUNCH	DINNER	SNACKS

WATER: ☐☐☐☐☐☐☐☐   FEELINGS: ☺☺☺☹☹   SLEEP: ....   EXERCISE: ....
CRAVINGS/RESPONSE: ....
....

DAY 364

WEEKLY REFLECTIONS/NOTES

HOW DO YOU FEEL ABOUT HOW THIS WEEK WENT? WHAT CAN YOU DO TO
MAKE NEXT WEEK BETTER?

....
....
....
.... HABIT: .... / 7

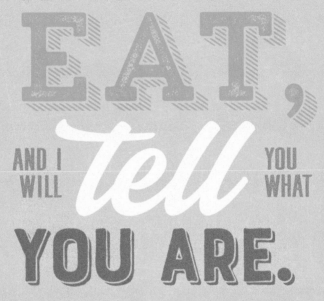

TELL ME WHAT YOU **EAT,** AND I WILL *tell* YOU WHAT **YOU ARE.**

–JEAN ANTHELME BRILLAT-SAVARIN

FINAL CHECK-IN

CURRENT MEASUREMENTS

WEIGHT: ....

UPPER ARMS: ....

CHEST: ....

WAIST: ....

HIPS: ....

THIGHS: ....

CALVES: ....

CONGRATULATIONS!

YOU'VE JUST FINISHED 52 WEEKS OF TAKING CHARGE OF YOUR
HEALTH AND WELLNESS!

HOW DO YOU FEEL ABOUT THE PAST FOUR WEEKS? DO YOU FEEL
YOU HAVE BEEN SUCCESSFUL MEETING YOUR GOALS?

....

....

....

....

....

....

....

....

....

....

....

....

....

....

....

....

....

....

ABOUT THE AUTHOR

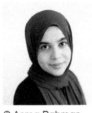

© Asma Rahman

NAZIMA QURESHI is a registered dietitian with a master of public health degree. She is the founder of Nutrition by Nazima, which has helped hundreds of women around the world transform their lives. Nazima helps others optimally nourish their bodies and improve their relationship with food without restrictive dieting. On any given day, she can be found reading to her kids, writing, seeing clients, or hosting a workshop. Nazima lives in Toronto, Canada, where she loves creating new recipes and spending time outdoors with her husband and two daughters.

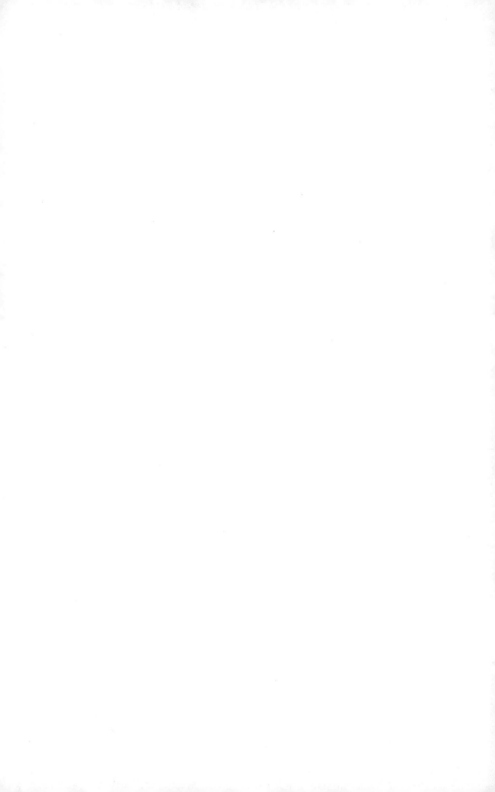

CPSIA information can be obtained
at www.ICGtesting.com
Printed in the USA
BVHW090459060819
555115BV00002B/2/P

9 781641 526258